MW01490080

ACLS PROVIDER MANUAL 2025 & EXAM PREP

Understand Advanced Cardiovascular Life Support and How to Pass ACLS Exam Using This Manual for Effective and Splendid Results

By

RUFUS LUCAS

Table of Contents

INTRODUCTION

ACLS certification is required for pre-med, medical, student, graduate, or practicing physician. So, it is essential that you prepare with necessary materials required to pass your certification exam in one sitting.

ACLS is an acronym for Advanced Cardiovascular Life Support or Advanced Cardiac Life Support which refer to the clinical algorithms used by healthcare professionals for urgent emergencies treatment.

Now that you're preparing to get certified in Advanced Cardiac Life Support, we have worked on gathering tips and study materials you need to pass the Certification Examination.

Emergencies ACLS is needed for

A good knowledge of Advanced Cardiovascular Life support is essential for healthcare professionals in order to attend to the following emergencies:

- Stroke
- Cardiac Arrest
- Myocardial Infarction
- Cardiovascular Emergencies

Your certification examination will include topics covering the emergencies listed above and will be discussed in

1

concluding sections of this book. You will also get preparatory questions and answers at the last section of the book.

And aside from topics relating to the ones listed above, the following are also essential:

- Care systems
- Team dynamics
- Acute dysthymia
- Team communication
- Immediate post cardiac arrest
- Acute coronary syndrome
- Recognition and intervention of cardiopulmonary arrest

ACLS certification and recertification is necessary for most healthcare professionals including nurses, doctors, firefighters, paramedics, emergency, and medical technicians.

ACLS UPDATED GUIDELINES

The advancement of medical knowledge and emergency response procedures is reflected in the history of Advanced Cardiac Life Support (ACLS), a major development in cardiac care. ACLS was developed by the American Heart Association (AHA) in 1974 to provide a standardized strategy for the urgent treatment of life-threatening cardiovascular emergencies such as cardiac arrest, stroke, and myocardial infarction.

ACLS has undergone multiple modifications since its establishment, each reflecting the growing body of clinical data and developing methods in cardiac care. The rules were updated in the 1980s and 1990s, most notably in 1980 and 1986, to reflect new research and technological advances. By 1992, the guidelines had expanded to include improved airway management techniques and pharmacological regimens.

These methods were refined further in the early 2000s. The modifications in 2000 and 2005 reflected a greater emphasis on early defibrillation and a broader role for non-physician healthcare personnel in providing ACLS. Subsequent modifications in 2010 and 2015 brought about major improvements, particularly in post-cardiac arrest treatment, airway management, and pharmaceutical use, as well as a greater emphasis on the significance of high-quality CPR and early intervention.

The 2020 upgrade marked a watershed moment. ACLS underwent a major redesign this year to better coincide with the International Liaison Committee on Resuscitation (ILCOR) recommendations. This revision broke with the customary five-year cycle of revisions, moving to an online model that allowed for more regular changes. This change allowed for a more dynamic and flexible guideline approach, ensuring healthcare practitioners access the most up-to-date evidence-based practices.

ACLS has had a significant impact on healthcare and patient outcomes. The guidelines have become important to medical, nursing, and paramedical education and have influenced resuscitation protocols worldwide. Over the years, the evolution of ACLS has greatly improved outcomes in cardiac arrest and other cardiovascular emergencies. Early intervention, high-quality CPR, and post-resuscitation care have increased survival rates and improved patient outcomes. Furthermore, incorporating technology improvements, such as AEDs, upgraded airway devices, and improved pharmaceutical therapies, has increased the efficiency of ACLS.

In essence, ACLS history is a story of ongoing development and adaptability in the face of growing medical knowledge. The move to an online, constantly updated format demonstrates a modern approach to medical guideline development, highlighting the need for agility and responsiveness to new evidence and technologies in emergency cardiovascular care.

Advanced interventional protocols and algorithms for treating cardiopulmonary emergencies like myocardial infarction, cardiac arrest, tachycardias, bradycardias, and stroke are included in the 2023 Advanced Cardiac Life Support (ACLS) recommendations. The following are key components of the guidelines:

Secondary ABCD (Airway, Breathing, Circulation, Differential Diagnosis)

The ACLS standards' Secondary ABCD method includes key measures for dealing with emergencies, with a special emphasis on sustaining vital functions:

- **Airway Management:** Airway Management entails ensuring that the patient's airway is clear and unobstructed for effective breathing. To deliver rescue breaths, healthcare practitioners are advised to utilize an Ambu bag and a mask with full-flow oxygen. The airway's patency (openness) must be monitored continuously to remain clear throughout treatment.

- **Breathing:** It is critical to ensure the patient's breathing is effective. During this stage, healthcare providers must monitor and manage the patient's breathing pattern and effectiveness and look for signs of respiratory distress or failure.

- **Circulation:** This stage entails evaluating and assisting the patient's blood circulation. Monitoring heart rate and rhythm, blood pressure, and oxygenation are all part of it. Medication, fluids, or other therapies may be administered as interventions to maintain appropriate circulation and blood pressure.

- **Differential Diagnosis:** This is how healthcare providers assess multiple probable reasons for a patient's ailment. This stage is critical for determining the underlying etiology of the emergency and guiding specific treatment measures.

It is critical to temporarily cease chest compressions while providing the two rescue breaths to allow for adequate ventilation without interference from compressions. This precise synchronization of breathing and compressions is critical for enhancing the effectiveness of resuscitation attempts.

Breathing

Confirming the precise installation of the advanced airway device is a critical step in Advanced Cardiac Life Support (ACLS) since it guarantees that the patient receives enough breathing and oxygenation. Several critical checks are performed during this process:

- **The Presence of Condensation in the Airway Device During Exhalation:** The presence of condensation in the airway device during exhalation is a simple yet effective indicator that the airway is in the respiratory tract and that air is going in and out.

- **Examining the Chest for Equal Bilateral Chest Rise:** This entails visually evaluating the chest to confirm that both sides of the chest rise evenly with each breath. Uneven chest rise may signal a problem, such as a pneumothorax, or that the airway device is not adequately positioned in the trachea.

- **Auscultating for Equal Bilateral Breath Sounds:** Healthcare providers use a stethoscope to evaluate breath sounds on both sides of the chest. This helps establish that air enters both lungs equally and that the airway device is neither blocked nor dislodged.

- **Ensure that no esophageal intubation has occurred:** Esophageal intubation occurs when an airway device is accidentally placed into the esophagus rather than the trachea. This is a major mistake since it indicates that the patient is not being vented. Auscultation can assist in detecting this since breath sounds will not be present in the lungs, and instead, stomach noises may be heard.

- **End-tidal CO2 (EtCO2) Monitoring:** Monitoring end-tidal CO2 levels is critical for ensuring successful breathing and airway device installation. Continuous monitoring of EtCO2 is advised in patients with an advanced airway in place. A capnography or EtCO2 monitor can provide real-time feedback on the patient's exhaled CO2 levels. An abrupt drop or lack of EtCO2 can suggest an airway device problem, such as dislodgement or obstruction.

These tests are essential to the ACLS protocol because they ensure that oxygen is delivered to the patient effectively, which is critical for preserving key organ function during a cardiopulmonary emergency. The objective is to quickly identify and rectify airway device problems to improve patient outcomes.

Circulation

The regulation of circulation is a vital component of Advanced Cardiac Life Support (ACLS). This step consists of numerous critical actions:

- **How to Get Intravenous (IV) or Intraosseous (IO) Access:** It is critical to establish a dependable route for the delivery of drugs and fluids. IV access is usually the initial option, although IO access (straight into the bone marrow) is an option if IV access is not possible. This access enables the immediate introduction of life-saving medications and fluids into circulation.
- **Monitoring with Various equipment:** Assessing and maintaining the patient's circulatory state requires various monitoring equipment.

These are some examples:
- **Electrocardiogram (ECG):** It offers critical information about the electrical activity of the heart and aids in the identification of certain cardiac rhythms, which is necessary for directing proper treatment.
- **Blood Pressure Cuff:** Blood pressure monitoring is critical for determining the effectiveness of the heart's pumping action and the patient's overall hemodynamic stability.
- **Pulse oximeter:** This non-invasive device detects the oxygen saturation of the patient's blood, providing instant feedback on the effectiveness of oxygen transport to the tissues.

- **End-Tidal CO2 (EtCO2) Monitor:** This device measures the quantity of carbon dioxide in exhaled air and can provide information about the patient's ventilation and circulation.

- **Heart Rhythm Identification:** Accurate heart rhythm identification is a cornerstone of ACLS. This entails analyzing the ECG to determine the precise type of cardiac arrhythmia being experienced by the patient. Within the ACLS algorithms, each beat has its own set of potential treatments.

- **12-Lead ECG:** Obtaining a 12-lead ECG can provide more detailed data about the heart's electrical activity and aid in diagnosing certain disorders such as myocardial infarction.

- **Initiating Appropriate Therapy:** Specific therapeutic measures are initiated based on the determined cardiac rhythm. Drug therapy, electrical therapy (such as defibrillation, cardioversion, or pacing), and other supportive measures may be used. Each ECG-identified cardiac rhythm has a related ACLS treatment algorithm that guides healthcare providers in providing the most effective and appropriate therapy.

This all-encompassing approach to circulation management is essential to ACLS because it strives to swiftly restore and sustain adequate circulatory function, critical for patient survival and recovery in cardiac crises.

Differential Diagnosis

Differential diagnosis is critical in ACLS, especially when considering reversible causes of rhythm/arrhythmia. This procedure entails a comprehensive examination to determine the underlying cause of the cardiac emergency, which is critical for determining the best course of treatment. Typically, the strategy entails:

- **Assessing Hypoxia:** Arrhythmias can be caused by low oxygen levels. The first step in treatment is to provide enough oxygenation.
- **Electrolyte Imbalances:** Electrolyte imbalances such as potassium, calcium, and magnesium can produce arrhythmias. It is critical to correct these imbalances.
- **Detecting Drug Toxicity or Overdose:** Arrhythmias can be caused by some drugs or toxic chemicals. Recognizing and managing medication toxicity is critical in patient care.

- **Acidosis testing:** Both metabolic and respiratory acidosis can cause alterations in heart rhythm. The underlying cause of acidosis can be treated to help stabilize the rhythm.
- **Evaluating Hypothermia:** A dangerously low body temperature might disrupt heart rhythm. Warmth and supportive treatment are critical.
- **Cardiac Tamponade:** This disorder, in which fluid accumulates around the heart, can result in arrhythmia. Immediate action is essential.
- **Taking Tension into Account Pneumothorax:** Due to increased pressure in the chest cavity, this potentially fatal disease can cause arrhythmia.
- **Evaluating for Thrombosis:** Arrhythmias can occur with both myocardial infarction (heart attack) and pulmonary embolism and require rapid treatment.
- **Assessing for Trauma:** Arrhythmias can be caused by traumatic injury to the heart or chest.

By systematically addressing these reversible reasons, healthcare providers can more precisely diagnose the underlying issue causing the arrhythmia and modify their treatment approach accordingly. This complete evaluation is critical for efficient cardiac emergency care and can greatly improve patient outcomes.

Cardiac/Electrical Therapy

In ACLS, cardiac/electrical therapy consists of many important interventions, each adapted to individual heart conditions:

- **Transcutaneous Pacemaker (TCP):** Used in persistent bradycardia that does not respond to medication. Bradycardia, or a sluggish heartbeat, can result in insufficient blood supply to the body. TCP uses pads and electrodes on the patient's chest to administer pacing impulses and offers temporary pacing through the skin. Pacing rates are often established to guarantee proper heart rate and rhythm, beginning at 60 beats per minute or slightly higher than the patient's intrinsic heart rate if measurable. TCP is critical in emergencies to keep cardiac output going until a more permanent solution is found.
- **Cardioversion:** Cardioversion is used when a patient has tachyarrhythmias (abnormally fast heart rhythms) such as Atrial Fibrillation, Atrial Flutter, Atrial Tachycardia, and Symptomatic Ventricular Tachycardia (VT). When medication therapy and

vagal maneuvers (techniques to reduce the heart rate) have failed, and the patient still has a pulse, cardioversion is indicated. A synchronized electrical shock is delivered to the heart at the same time as the R wave of the ECG to restore a normal rhythm. It is critical for stabilizing the patient's condition and avoiding consequences such as cardiac failure or stroke.

- **Defibrillation:** Defibrillation is a vital intervention for treating Ventricular Fibrillation (VF) along with pulseless Ventricular Tachycardia (VT), which are both life-threatening disorders in which the heart quivers or beats ineffectively. In certain circumstances, the heart is unable to adequately pump blood, resulting in a rapid collapse and cardiac arrest. Defibrillation delivers an unsynchronized high-energy shock to the heart to reset its electrical state and allow its natural pacemaker to re-establish an effective rhythm. Defibrillation efficiency declines with time, making it critical to perform during the first 5 minutes of cardiac arrest. CPR before and after the shock can improve defibrillation success by increasing blood flow to the heart and brain.

Each of these treatments is essential in the treatment of cardiac crises. The individual cardiac disease determines the therapy chosen, the patient's symptoms' severity, and the arrhythmia's underlying cause. The goal in all circumstances is to restore and maintain an appropriate heart rhythm and enough circulation, increasing the patient's chances of recovery. Frequently conducted in high-stakes, time-sensitive situations, these interventions necessitate qualified healthcare workers educated in ACLS protocols.

Bradycardia Treatment

Under ACLS standards, the approach to bradycardia treatment is modified based on the patient's stability and heart rate (below 60 bpm):

- **Monitoring in Stable Patients:** Continuous monitoring is required when a patient is hemodynamically stable but has a sluggish heart rate. This includes paying attention to the heart rate and rhythm, blood pressure, oxygen saturation, and overall clinical state. The idea is to spot any changes that could suggest a decline in the patient's condition.

- **Intervention in Unstable Patients:** Prompt treatment is essential when bradycardia causes hemodynamic instability. Poor perfusion, changed mental status, chest discomfort, hypotension, or evidence of shock are all symptoms of instability.

- **Epinephrine administration:** Epinephrine is frequently used as the first line of treatment in unstable bradycardia. It raises the heart rate and improves myocardial contractility, increasing cardiac output. The usual epinephrine dosage is 1mg IV every 3-5 minutes, as needed.

- Transcutaneous Pacing (TCP) is used if epinephrine fails to improve the patient's state or is regarded as immediately necessary. TCP uses external pads to send pacing impulses to the heart. It is a non-invasive technique for providing temporary pacing support until a more permanent method, such as transvenous pacing, can be established.

- **Transvenous Pacing:** This procedure includes inserting a pacing wire into the heart through a central vein, usually with fluoroscopic supervision. Compared to TCP, this approach provides more consistent and controlled pacing.

- **Alternative Drug Therapies:** Alternative drugs can be considered if TCP is ineffective or unavailable or

17

transvenous pacing is delayed. Two examples are dopamine, a vasopressor, and inotropic drug, and isoproterenol, a beta-agonist that elevates heart rate and myocardial contractility.

It is critical to reassess the patient's response to interventions throughout therapy constantly. The underlying cause of the bradycardia should be examined and, if found, treated. This holistic strategy guarantees that bradycardia patients receive quick and effective therapy, critical for preventing further worsening and improving outcomes.

Asystole Treatment

A major component of Advanced Cardiac Life Support (ACLS) is the treatment of asystole, a situation in which there is no visible electrical activity in the heart. The strategy entails the following steps:

- **Epinephrine administration:** Epinephrine is the major medication used to treat asystole. It stimulates the heart and raises blood pressure, which is essential without cardiac output. 1mg IV every 3-5 minutes is the recommended dose.

- Atropine is another medicine used in treating asystole, albeit its usefulness in this context is debatable. It is usually administered as 1mg IV every 3-5 minutes, with a maximum dose of 3mg. Atropine increases heart rate by inhibiting the parasympathetic functions of the heart.

- Continuing Cardiopulmonary Resuscitation (CPR): Effective CPR is critical in treating asystole. It ensures the circulation of oxygenated blood, transporting it to essential organs such as the brain and heart.

- Reversible Causes: Recognizing and treating reversible causes is critical. Considerations include hypoxia, hypothermia, acidosis, drug overdose, and electrolyte abnormalities.

- **Advanced Airway Management:** Asystole treatment includes establishing an efficient airway and providing appropriate oxygenation and ventilation.

Continuous ECG monitoring is vital for detecting any changes in heart rhythm. This systematic strategy seeks to reverse asystole and restore a viable heart rhythm, but it's vital to note that asystole is frequently associated with a bad prognosis. However, prompt and efficient application of these actions can boost survival odds.

Pulseless Electrical Activity

The following treatments are available for Pulseless Electrical Activity (PEA), a condition in which electrical activity is seen on the ECG but there is no effective heart pump function:

- **Epinephrine Administration:** The key medicine in PEA treatment is epinephrine, administered intravenously at 1mg every 3-5 minutes. Epinephrine acts as a vasoconstrictor during resuscitation, increasing coronary and cerebral blood flow.
- **Atropine for Bradycardic Rhythms:** If a bradycardic rhythm is detected in PEA, atropine can be injected. It's utilized to boost heart rate and cardiac output.
- **High-Quality CPR:** It is critical to provide high-quality CPR consistently. It maintains blood circulation to vital organs.
- **Identify and Treat Reversible Causes:** Finding and treating reversible causes is an important element of PEA management. Look for hypoxia, hypovolemia, hydrogen ion (acidosis), hypo/hyperkalemia, hypothermia, toxins, cardiac tamponade, tension

pneumothorax, thrombosis (coronary or pulmonary), and trauma.

- **Advanced Airway Management:** Ensuring correct airway management and enough oxygenation is critical.

This method seeks to restore effective cardiac output while treating the underlying causes of PEA.

Acute Stroke

Acute stroke therapy within the scope of Advanced Cardiac Life Support (ACLS) guidelines necessitates a thorough and time-sensitive approach:

- **Immediate Assessment and Intervention:** The patient's cardiac rhythm should be checked within 10 minutes of presentation in the emergency room, and any arrhythmias should be addressed according to the ACLS algorithms. This is critical since cardiac comorbidities are widespread in stroke patients and can hurt the prognosis.
- **Early Neurological Evaluation:** A rapid neurological evaluation is required to establish the

stroke's severity and make key decisions about future therapy. This includes assessing the patient's state of consciousness and their capacity to communicate, understand, and move.

- **Imaging Studies:** A non-contrast CT scan of the head should be performed as soon as possible (preferably within 25 minutes of arrival) to differentiate between ischemic and hemorrhagic stroke, as the therapy for each differs dramatically. The scan can tell whether there is any bleeding in the brain, which would rule out some treatments, such as thrombolytic.

- **Regarding Fibrinolytic Therapy:** If the patient is a candidate and the onset of stroke symptoms is less than 3 hours (up to 4.5 hours in some situations), fibrinolytic therapy (usually intravenous alteplase) should be investigated. The goal of this treatment is to break the blood clot that is causing the ischemic stroke, restoring blood flow to the damaged part of the brain.

- **Exclusion of Contraindications:** Before delivering fibrinolytic therapy, any contraindications such as recent surgery, bleeding disorders, or a history of hemorrhagic stroke must be ruled out.

- **Supportive Care and Monitoring:** It is critical to continuously check vital signs, oxygenation, and blood glucose levels. Blood pressure control, fever management, and hyperglycemia treatment are examples of supportive care.
- **Further Interventions:** Mechanical thrombectomy (clot removal via a catheter) may be possible for certain ischemic strokes, particularly those affecting big blood vessels if conducted within a defined time limit from symptom start.
- **Rehabilitation and Complication Prevention:** Early therapy and steps to avoid complications like deep vein thrombosis are critical parts.

This all-encompassing approach to acute stroke therapy in the emergency setting is critical for reducing brain damage and improving outcomes. Emergency medicine, neurology, radiology, and other ancillary services must work together to provide prompt and effective care.

These updated guidelines include detailed strategies to help healthcare workers address a variety of acute cardiac and stroke crises.

24

ACLS STUDY TIPS

The tips listed below will help greatly in passing your certification examination with ease.

Get familiar with situations where ACLS is needed, and procedures involved

While you prepare for your certification examination, be mindful of importance of getting familiar with the practical aspect of the course. Review different cases where ACLS is needed and the symptoms and procedures involved, do this before your certification examination.

Your certification is evidence that you possess the professional skills needed to partake in medical activities relating to Advanced Cardiac Life Support. When you're not yet certified to partake in the practical aspect, you can review the practical process. Therefore, reviewing more practical aspects helps more in the theoretical aspects of the course.

Study ACLS Algorithms as Early as Possible

ACLS algorithms are flowcharts of procedures required to treat certain situations where ACLS is needed. It is better to learn these algorithms early before your test so you can get your own unique style of memorizing them.

Algorithms to learn for your certification examination are:

- Acute Coronary Syndromes (ACS) algorithm
- Adult BLS Algorithm
- Adult bradycardia algorithm
- Adult cardiac arrest algorithm
- Adult suspected stroke algorithm
- Adult tachycardia algorithm immediate post-cardiac arrest care algorithm
- Opioid-associated life-threatening emergency algorithm
- Unstable tachycardia algorithm

Memorize medications needed for certain situations

These are best prepared for by creating mnemonic flashcards. Parts of the certification examination questions will include identifying medications and dosages needed for different medical ACLS situations. Giving a wrong medication may be bad for the outcome of the examination. Therefore, review different medications required for different situations where ACLS is needed. Start studying them as early as possible so you can cover all the aspects you have to cover.

Understand the different causes that may lead to patients' situation

This is essential to pass your exam. Its shows your knowledge of the ACLS algorithms. These are categorized into two (Hs and Ts) and are best memorized with mnemonic devices.

The Hs and Ts include the following:

- Hypoxia
- Hypovolemia
- Hydrogen ion (acidosis)
- Hyper or Hypokalemia (Potassium)

- Hypothermia

- Toxins

- Tension Pneumothorax

- Tamponade (Pericardial Tamponade)

- Thrombosis (Pulmonary Embolus)

- Thrombosis (Acute Coronary Syndrome)

Understand basic electrocardiography

Electrocardiography measures electrical activities of the heartbeat. This is done by placing electrodes on the patient's skin to record the activity on the graph.

Electrocardiography (EKG) must be understood in order to pass your ACLS exam. Further details on EKG have been discussed in further parts of this book.

Brace yourself up with practice exams

Gather enough questions and practice exams you can test yourself with in order to be familiarized with the exam you anticipate. Practice exam questions and answers have been added at the end of this book to further expand your knowledge and give you a clue of the kind of questions you should be prepared for.

ACLS EXAM TIPS

This is the part when you're seated for your exam. The former tips which were discussed earlier are essential before the exam starts while the ones that will be discussed now are useful during the exam.

Unlike the study tips, you now have a shorter time to showcase your preparations and how well you've study. Therefore, a shorter time in this case means fewer actions.

- All questions must be read thoroughly and understood in a view to give the correct answers to the questions which are always technical and misreading the questions increases the chances of coming up with wrong answers.

- You'll be given a period to answer all questions and you don't want to waste most of the time given puzzling over the hard questions you first approach. Therefore, skip the hard questions and go for the simpler ones first and once you're done, you can go for the difficult ones. This method makes you answer more questions within a shorter period without being stressed out.

- Don't be anxious about the exam, be calm. The tips above as well as the concluding parts of this book are good enough to get you prepared for the examination.

A SUMMARY OF TYPES OF DEVICES USED TO PROVIDE SUPPLEMENTARY OXYGEN AND THEIR FUNCTIONS

It is important that people suffering from acute coronary syndrome, pulmonary diseases, stroke or other life-threatening diseases be, at frequent intervals, administered oxygen. Administering oxygen is such an important and life-saving task that different devices have been invented to make this task simple and effective.

Types of Devices Used to Provide Supplementary Oxygen

Devices used in providing supplementary oxygen include:

- Venturi Mask

- Simple Oxygen Face Mask

- Nasal Cannula

- Face Mask with Oxygen Reservoir

It is important to ascertain the working conditions of these devices before, during and after using them to administer oxygen to patients, in order to avoid fatal errors.

Oxygen Supply

Oxygen Supply is an important factor in administering Oxygen. It simply refers the cylinder or wall unit connecting a patient to the oxygen administering device; it delivers oxygen from the device to the patient. To ensure that the Oxygen Supply to the patient is optimal and functioning, you'd have to crosscheck the following equipment.

- The tubing system that connects the patient's oxygen administering equipment to the patient.

- The Valve handles that open the cylinder.

- Pressure Gauge

- Flow Meter; and

- The Oxygen Administration device itself.

Note additionally, to ensure a seamless oxygen administration process, that it must be administered by a trained individual.

It is quite enough to be trained as an advanced cardiovascular provider. This advanced training must include in-depth knowledge of the emergency usage of the equipment just in case the need arises.

Simple Oxygen Face Mask

This device administers low-flow oxygen to the patient's mouth and nose. At the rate of about 6 to 10 L/min, this device can supply up to 60% oxygen; though the ultimate oxygen concentration depends largely on how the mask is fit on the patient, see table 1 for more information. For this device to be effectively used, to prevent the rebreathing of exhaled carbon dioxide (CO_2) and to maintain an increase in the inhalation of oxygen concentration, this device needs to have the least flow rate of 6 L/min.

Venturi Mask

This Oxygen-administering device allows more concentrated oxygen, about 24% to 60% more to be administered to the patient. Using a flow rate of 8 L/min, the level of concentrated oxygen this device delivers can be adjusted to 24%, 28%, 35% and 40%. For a level of 40% to 50%, a flow rate of 10 to 12 l/min is used.

Respiratory depression is a common side-effect of this device. Patients must be frequently observed to prevent this, and also to avoid shunting. The oximeter must be utilized quickly to set the device to the preferred level of concentrated oxygen to be administered to the patient, as the situation demands.

This device is particularly useful for patients suffering from Chronic Obstructive Pulmonary Disease (COPD), Chronic Hypercarbdia (high CO_2), and mild to moderate hypoxemia, because it can accurately control the level of concentrated oxygen that is delivered to the patients at varying times.

Though patients with COPD can suffer from respiratory depression when high concentrated oxygen is administered to them due to a spike in PaO2 which eliminated the stimulant effect of hypoxemic on the respiratory centers, oxygen shouldn't be withdrawn from such patients. Instead, ventilation is supported, in cases of hypoxic ventilator drive.

Nasal Cannula

The Nasal Cannula is usually regarded as a low-flow administration system designed to administer oxygen to the room air that the patient inhales. The cannula's flow rate, alongside the depth and frequency at which the client breathes, determines the oxygen concentration while administering oxygen. Despite these two factors, the Nasal

Cannula can provide up to 44% oxygen mixed with room air. Inhalation of concentration oxygen to approximately 4% can be achieved by increasing the oxygen flow by 1 L/min. Note that the Oxygen flow has a starting limit of 1 L/min and a maximum limit of 6 L/min.

Recently, new research into high-flow variations of Nasal Cannula has shown interesting result. It's being reported that high-flow nasal cannula allows oxygen flow rate up to 60 L/min, sometimes exceeding this value. This can make patient inhale oxygen concentrated air of up to 100%.

For Nasal Cannula device to be effective, the patient must have airway protective mechanism, tidal volume, and adequate spontaneous respiratory effort.

Nasal Cannula is best used for patients:

✓ With Arterial oxyhemoglobin saturation less than 94%; less than 90% for patients suffering from Acute Coronary Syndromes (ACS)

✓ Who cannot tolerate the irritation of face mask.

✓ With minor respiratory or oxygenation problems.

Face Mask with Oxygen Reservoir

The face mask, as shown below in Fig. 1, is a facial rebreathing mask. It usually comes with a medical face mask that's attached to an oxygen reservoir bag. This device provides up to 95% to 100% concentrated oxygen with a flow rate of 10 to 15 L/min, as seen in table 1. The device works effectively as a constant flow of oxygen reservoir goes through the facial rebreathing mask to the patient.

This device is recommended to patients who are critically ill with spontaneous breathing, though they have adequate tidal volume but require high concentrated oxygen to be administered to them. Patients with Acute Pulmonary Edeme, COPD or Asthma would want to avoid Endotracheal (ET) intubation as it might inflame their lungs.

Additionally, patients who are being readied for advance airway management, or have indications for advanced airway management but maintain gags, coughs, or another airway protective reflexive, are advised to use this device.

Using this device also comes with its own risks. Patients might experience diminished consciousness level, or experience nausea and/or vomiting. In cases where the device is closely fitted to the patient, incessant monitoring is required, and suctioning devices must be within easy reach.

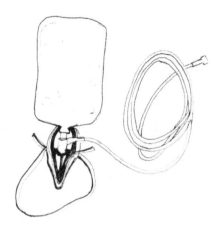

Figure 1: Face Mask with Oxygen Reservoir

Mouth-to-Mouth Breaths for Adult Patients

If a health worker intends to give an adult patient Mouth-to-Mouth breathing with a Pocket Mask, he/she must be positioned beside the patient's side, especially when the health worker is performing a 1-rescuer cardiopulmonary resuscitation (CPR). This would enable the health worker to give breaths and perform chest compressions simultaneously without having to change positions. Using a pocket mask to give mouth-to-mouth might be tricky, but following these practical steps would make it easier. Remember that a patient suspected to have neck or spinal cord complications must be in a head-tilt, chin-lift maneuver to allow effective breath giving.

i.   Perch yourself firmly by the side of the patient.

ii.   Use the bridge of the nose to correctly guide you in placing the pocket mask on the patient's face.

iii.   Seal the pocket mask against the face

iv.   Place your thumb and index finger along the edge of the mask, preferably the hand the nearest to the patient's head is advised.

v.   Place the thumb of your other hand along the edge of the mask.

vi.   Use a head-tilt, chin-lift to open the airway and place your remaining fingers of your other hand along the bony margin of the jaw, lifting the jaw in the process. This process is shown clearly in Fig. 2.

vii.   Press firmly on both the lifted jaw and the edge of the mask to firmly seal the pocket mask against the patients face and prevent air from escaping.

viii.   Each breath is administered over 1 second, long enough to make the patient's chest rise.

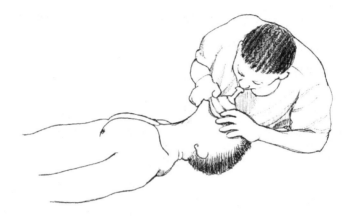

Figure 2: Mouth-to-Mouth Breaths for Adult Patients

Bag-Mask Ventilation

This oxygen administering device comprises of a self-inflating bag and a non-rebreathing valve. It can be conjoined with face mask or used as an advanced airway management. The mask in this device must be tight sealed on the face, covering both mouth and nose in order to be effective. Additionally, in order to be able track, the regurgitation of patient, the mask must be transparent.

This device is especially useful for patients who suffer difficulty in breathing since it administers high concentrated oxygen to them, and comes in different ranges of sizes, from infants to adults. Some of these devices are designed to allow positive and-expiratory pressure valve to be added to the structure.

Using this device correctly and effectively requires a certain level competency. For easy administration, it is advised that health workers work together to administer oxygen to the patients with this device. When one health worker opens the airway and seals the mask against the patient's nose and mask, the other gently and periodically squeezes the bag, as they both watch for visible chest rise.

Well-trained health workers can use this device to administer room air or oxygen if they utilize a self-inflating bag. If used without an advanced airway, this device provides positive-pressure ventilation which may produce gastric inflation and some other complications in different patients.

Important Cautions to Take While Performing a Bag-Mask Ventilation

✓ It is advised to, as soon as possible, insert an oropharyngeal airway into the patient to keep the airway open, providing the patient has no cough or gag reflex.

✓ When it comes to using a Bag-Mask Ventilation, it is strongly advised that two well-trained and experienced health workers use this device together on a patient.

✓ For Bag-Mask Ventilation to be effective, a leak-proof mask seal must be achieved. To achieve this, the health care worker would have to perform a head-tilt on the patient, and then maintain it with the use of his/her thumb and index finger to make a "C" shape, pressing the edged of the mask tightly against the face. The remaining fingers are then used to lift the angle of the jaw and open the airway. For this mask seal to be effective, the hand holding the mask against the face must be able to perform simultaneous tasks, i.e. maintain the head-tilt while pressing the mask firmly against the face, and lifting the jaw in the process.

✓ The use of an advanced airway device with the Bag-Mask device, like laryngeal mask airway, laryngeal tube, esophageal-tracheal tube (ET tube) etc., prevents any seal and/or volume problem from occurring.

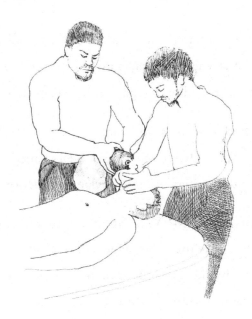

Figure 3: Bag-Mask Ventilation

Use of Advanced Airway and Chest Compression Method in Providing Ventilation

Using an advanced airway during CPR is commendable, but it also comes with some precaution. When a patient is placed on an advanced airway device during CPR, it is imperative to continually provide compressions and asynchronous ventilation once every 6 seconds.

Furthermore, rescuers must avoid excessive ventilation i.e., too many breaths or too large a volume.

ADVANCED AIRWAY
MANAGEMENT

Members of an Advanced Airway

The advanced airway is made up of different members including:

- The laryngeal tube
- The laryngeal mask airway and
- Esophageal-tracheal tube

Laryngeal tube

The Laryngeal tube, as seen in Fig. 4, is a supraglottic airway. This device is commonly considered as a substitute to an ET tube. You can find this device in both single and dual-lumen versions. The usage of this is quite tricky so only professional and experienced health care workers should perform an insertion with it.

This device comes with some certain advantages though. Some of them are:

- Due to its compact size, the device allows ease of training and insertion.

- When compared to bag-mask ventilation, Laryngeal tube actually isolates the airway of the patient, hence, leading to decreased risk of aspiration and provides reliable ventilation.

- This device is also preferred, by numerous trained health workers, to bag-mask ventilation or ET because of its efficient airway management in patients with cardiac arrest.

  Insertion of the Laryngeal tube:

✓ Prepare Patients by providing adequate oxygenation and ventilation, and also positioning the patients optimally.

✓ In the same way, check and double-check the integrity of the Laryngeal tube, making sure all is complete and functional in consonance with the manufacturer's instruction.

✓ Inspect both the mouth of the patient and the larynx of the patient to ensure there is no blockage.

✓ Use the thumb-and-index-finger technique to open the mouth of the patient to about 2-3cm.

✓ Gently insert the Laryngeal tube in the midline of the mouth along the palate. Stop when you feel a slight resistance.

✓ Slight head extension can, in some cases, enable ease of mouth opening and also help tube placement.

✓ Ensure that the Ventilation holes of the larynx align in front of the Laryngeal Inlet.

✓ The teeth marks at the upper end of the tube determine how deep the insertion of the device would be.

✓ The Laryngeal tube comes in different sizes, so be sure to use the appropriate size for each patient.

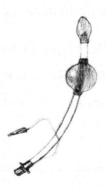

Figure 4: The laryngeal tube

The Laryngeal Mask Airway

This device, as shown in fig. 5, consists of a tube with a cuffed, mask-like projection at its end. This device is an advanced airway management device that's also considered as a very good alternative to ET tube. During CPR, laryngeal mask airway, when compared to other airway devices like the ET tube, provides ventilation of about 72% to 97% of patients. It is important for health worker to have a back-up strategy or device for airway management since Laryngeal mask airway cannot ventilate a small portion of patients.

Despite this setback, this device had the following advantages:

- The risk of Regurgitation is decreased with this device than bag-mask device

- Training for Laryngeal mask airway insertion is not as complex or strenuous, as compared to ET intubation, since it does not require laryngoscopy and visualization of the cords.

- In cases where access to the patient is limited due the possibility of unstable neck injury, or positioning patients for ET intubation is physically impossible, laryngeal mask airway is much easier and safer.

Steps to follow to insert the Laryngeal Mask Airway into the patients as illustrated in fig. 6:

- Prepare the patient to provide optimum oxygenation and ventilation through proper positioning

- Check the Integrity of both the mask and tube and ensure that they function properly in adherence to the manufacturer's instruction. Lubricating only the posterior surface of the cuff would avoid blocking the airway aperture.

- Slowly insert the Laryngeal mask into the Pharynx until you feel resistance. This resistance means that the tube had reached the hypopharynx

- Cuff Inflation pushes the mask up against the trachea opening which allows air to flow freely through the tube and into the trachea; so, ensure to inflate the cuff of the mask

- This device delivers oxygen through the tube which does so by administering oxygen to the opening of the center of the mask, and directly into the trachea.

- Gently and slowly the laryngeal mask airway into the patient's mouth, and no occasion must force be used in order to avoid trauma.

- Be careful not to overinflate the cuff as this can lead to excessive intracuff pressure which may result in misplacement of the device. It could also cause pharyngolaryngeal injury such as sore throat, dysphagia or nerve injury.

- Use bite-block in cases there the laryngeal mask airway is not designed with one. Bite-block provides ventilation to the patient, and it also enable the health worker to adequately monitor both the patient's condition and the position of the laryngeal mask airway. A bite block also decreases the chances of airway obstruction and/or tube damage.

- Ensure you keep the bite-block in place until you completely remove the laryngeal mask airway from the patient's mouth.

In order to ensure the smooth success of using the Laryngeal mask airway on the patient, some additional information should be adhered to. Some of them are:

- Do not apply cricoid pressure. Doing this may prevent the ease and complete insertion of the laryngeal mask airway. Research has shown that when cricoid pressure is used before insertion of the laryngeal mask airway, the rate at which the tube is correctly positioned reduces greatly, and also increases the rate of failed insertion and impaired ventilation when the Laryngeal mask airway is finally inserted.

- Since there are different sizes of this device, size 5 generally fits men while size 4 usually fits women, though this may differ in some situations.

- Sometimes, there may appear on the patient's cricoid cartilage a smooth swelling. This is quite normal as it indicates the proper positioning of the device.

- Ensure to reevaluate the position of the laryngeal mask airway if you hear air leak during ventilation for about 3 to 4 breaths, in order to avoid possible misplacement.

- Another means of avoiding possible misplacement is to restrict the movement of the patient's head, and also avoid suctioning secretions in the pharynx once the laryngeal mask airways has been fully inserted.

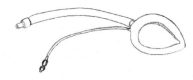

Figure 5: The laryngeal mask airway

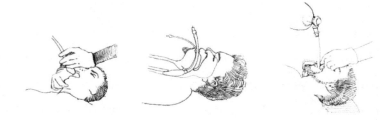

Figure 6: Inserting the laryngeal mask airway

Esophageal-Tracheal Tube

The esophageal-tracheal tube, as shown in fig. 7, is an advanced airway management device, and also a great alternative to ET intubation. This device is an invasive airway device designed with 2 inflatable balloon cuffs. The tube is designed to easily enter the esophagus rather than the trachea, which means ventilation through the side openings of the device which is placed adjacent to the vocal cords and trachea. If the tube is inserted through the trachea, ventilation can still occur by an opening in the end of the tube.

Different research carried out has shown that different level of healthcare workers, regardless of their experience, can effectively use the esophageal-tracheal tube to effectively administer and manage airway ventilation in patients as comparable to ET intubation which requires high level of expertise.

Furthermore, when compared to Bag-mask ventilation, the esophageal-tracheal tube holds better advantage because it does a better job at isolating the patient's airway, decrease the risk of aspiration, and enabled effective and efficient ventilation. Though, Esophageal-tracheal tube has the advantage of ease of training for health workers over ET intubation, only experience and trained should use the device.

Misuse could lead to fatal complications, especially if the distal lumen of the device in the esophagus or trachea is identified incorrectly.

Other possible complications associated with using the esophageal tracheal tube include:

—   Esophageal trauma

—   Lacerations

—   Bruising; and

—   Subcutaneous emphysema.

The Esophageal tube is designed in 2 sizes. The smaller of the sizes is 37ft, and it is used for patients that are 4 to 5.5 feet tall, while the larger size is 41F which is used for patients that are more than 5 feet tall.

Contraindications

—   Patients that have are sensitive to insertion and react with cough or gag reflex

—   Patients that are 16 years or younger

—   Patients that are 4 feet or shorter.

—   Recognized or suspected esophageal disease

–   Patients that have ingested caustic substance.

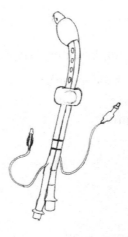

Figure 7: The esophageal tracheal tube

Practical step-by-step guide to Insert Esophageal-Tracheal Tube

Step 1: Same way with other devices, you prepare the patient for oxygenation and ventilation by properly positioning the patient. Health workers should rule out the contraindications to insertion of this device.

Step 2: Ensure you go over the safety and effectiveness of the equipment multiple times, to make sure it corresponds with manufacturer's regulations before commencing with the operation. Also ensure that the tube is well lubricated.

Step 3: To properly insert the esophageal tube:

-   Ensure you hold the esophageal tube with the deflated cuff which would ensure that the curvature of the tube aligns well with curvature of the pharynx.

-   Gently lift the jaw and insert the tube slowly until the black lines are positioned between the patient's upper teeth. never force the device into the patient's throat and do not attempt for more than 30 seconds.

-   Inflate the Proximal/pharyngeal and 10 cuff with 100 ml of air. For the smaller sized esophageal-tracheal tube, inflate with 85 ml. After that, you would inflate the distal with air of 15ml, and 12ml for smaller sized esophageal-tracheal tube.

Step 4: Ascertain the location of the tube then carefully select the lumen for adequate ventilation. In order to correctly select the appropriate Lumen, you must ascertain where the tip is exactly located, which could only lie either at the esophagus or the trachea.

Step 5: You would need to confirm the placement of the esophagus by attaching the bag-mask to the proximal/laryngeal. When you squeeze the bag, you provide ventilation the patient by forcing air through the openings in the tube which lies between the two inflated cuffs. This squeezing action produce what is often called bilateral sound. Epigastric sounds do not occur because, once the distal cuff is inflated, it obstructs the esophagus, thereby prevent air from flowing into the stomach. Due to the simple fact that the distal tube, labeled white rests solely in the esophagus, do not use it for ventilation.

Step 6: If breathing sounds do not occur after squeezing the bag attached to the proximal/laryngeal, disconnect the bag immediately and reattach it to the distal lumen. When this is done, squeezing the bag should now produce breath sounds because this lumen connects straight to the trachea. In ET tube placement, the distal cuff performs the same function as a cuff on an ET tube. Detection of exhaled CO_2 (through the ventilating lumen) should be used for confirmation, particularly if the patient has a perfusing rhythm.

Step 7: If the breathing sounds don't occur or you're unable to hear it, then you should deflate both cuffs and slightly withdraw the tube. Check the previous steps to re-inflate both cuffs and ventilate the patient again. If breath sounds and epigastric sounds still don't occur, then remove the tube. Ensure there is suction equipment within reach just in case removal of the tube causes vomiting.

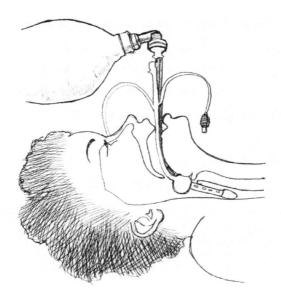

Figure 8: Inserting the esophageal tracheal tube

Other relevant information to this device include:

– Applying Cricoid pressure on the patient during insertion is big No. Due to the fact the pressure may hinder the insertion of the esophageal-tracheal tube.

The downsides of choosing Esophageal-tracheal tube over other means of airflow management are:

- Insertion of this device may lead to esophageal trauma in some patients. These traumas include lacerations, bruising, and subcutaneous emphysema.

- This device is only manufactured in two sizes and cannot be used in any patient less than 4 feet tall.

ET Intubation

An ET tube is an airway management device used to administer high concentration of energy and selected tidal volume to maintain adequate ventilation in patients. This is device is designed to be for a single-use and comes with a cuffed tube. The placement of this device demands that the health worker or rescuer is able to clearly visualize the patient's vocal cords.

The advantages of ET tube Insertion are:

- It allows for the effective suctioning of the trachea

- It serves as very effective viable alternative for delivering resuscitation medications to patients when Intraosseous (IO) or Intravenous (IV) access is restricted

- It maintains Patent Airway

- The ET tube is ideal for long term ventilation

- It could protect the airway from foreign substances, such as aspiration from stomach contents or other materials in the mouth, throat or nose.

- It effectively enables the administering of positive end-expiratory pressure.

- When the situation of the patient is quite critical and required higher degree of airway pressure, ET tube is the device to use.

- ET tube is compatible with many drugs that could be administered to the patient through it. such drugs include atropine, naloxone, epinephrine, and lidocaine.

  For drug administration, ET tube has the following head-start.

- ET tube allows, if need be, a higher dosage of drugs of about 2 to 2.5 times higher than IV or IO administration.

- For better drug absorption, mix the dosage of the drug with about 5ml to 10ml to pure saline or sterile water. It has been shown through series of research that when drugs like epinephrine and lidocaine are diluted with sterile water instead of 0.9 saline solution, a better drug absorption is achieved.

- To ensure effective and complete facilitation of the drug throughout the whole system of the patient, the health worker should perform one or two ventilations on the patient after the drug has been delivered through the ET tube.

- During instillation of drugs into the patient through the ET tube, briefly hold chest compressions on the patient. This is done because chest compressions will enable contents of the drug to come back out of the ET tube in cases where the bag-mask device is not reconnected, so as to prevent fatal complications when the drug is not properly circulated through the system of the patient.

Though ET tube has some advantages when it comes to administering drugs to patients, IV/IO administration is preferred. This is because the optimal method of administering drug through ET tube is yet to be fully determined and IV/IO provides a more reliable means of delivering drug to meet the required pharmacologic effect.

Some individuals had argued the case of ET tube as the optimal means of ventilating the airway during cardiac arrest, but the vast degree of fatal complications that can occur if an unskilled health worker attempts intubation with the ET tube has been inimical to the argument. This has led to the emergence of esophageal-tracheal tubes, laryngeal mask airways, and laryngeal tubes to be accepted as effective alternatives to ET tube which is, all things considered, more advanced than other ways of advanced airway management.

Since a slight misplacement of ET tube can lead to critical, sometimes fatal, complications, only experienced and highly skilled health workers perform ET intubation. Most states that practice medical acts actually specify the level or rank of personnel that are allowed to carry out ET intubation. In cases where the ET tube is to be used for clinical reasons, only health workers who have met these criteria should use the ET tube:

- They must be well-trained

- They must perform ET tube intubations at frequent intervals

- They must go through regular refresher-training regarding ET tube intubation in order to sharpen their skills.

- Placement of ET tube is included in the scope of practice as stipulated by the government.

- They must regularly participate in quality improvement process in order to detect the complications that are most common and how to guard against it.

Although the placement of the ET tube during a resuscitation attempt is important, frequent, high-quality and effective chest compressions coupled with few interruptions and swift delivery of defibrillation is more important.

To Give an Effective ET Intubation, the Following Cautions Must Be Adhered to:

Although most health workers don't practice the use of ET tube intubation due to the reasons explained above and the high standards it requires, it is pertinent for all health workers to at least understand how the process of ET tube intubation works. Health workers may work in teams to integrate compressions and ventilation when the ET tube is placed. Knowing the process, sometimes, is more important than actually knowing how to perform the procedure itself.

Step 1: Considering the patient's anatomy, decide the optimal position through which the patient would receive optimum oxygenation and ventilation.

Step 2: Assemble and cross-check the parts that make up the ET tube and ascertain their integrity.

Step 3: Choosing the appropriate size of ET tube for the patient comes next. Usually, a 7.5 to 8.00 mm internal diameter is used for male adult, and a 7.0 to 7.5mm internal diameter is used for female adults.

Step 4: Use the appropriate type, either straight or curved, and the appropriate size of the laryngoscope blade.

Step 5: Ensure you test the ET tube cuff's integrity.

Step 6: Secure the stylet and lubricate the ET tube

Step 7: Place the head in the sniffing position, and, using the thumb-and-index-finger technique, open the mouth of the patient.

Step 8: If necessary, clear the airway, then slowly insert the laryngoscope blade while visualizing the glottic opening.

Step 9: Insert the ET tube through the vocal cords then inflate the ET tube cuff in order to achieve an effective seal.

Step 10: Remove the laryngoscope blade from the patient's mouth and hold the tube with one hand while removing the stylet with the other; after which you insert a bite shock.

Step 11: Attach an airbag to the tube and squeeze to give breath, one seconds per squeeze, while watching keenly for the chest to rise.

Step 12: Check for:

– Using auscultation, check for breath sounds

– Ensure the position of the ET tube is correct by performing a continuous quantitative waveform capnography or, if not within reach, a qualitative partial-pressure end-tidal CO_2 (PETCO$_2$), or esophageal detector device (EDD).

Step 13: Use the tube holder, or any other means, to secure the ET tube in position.

Step 14: Continue to deliver oxygen and monitor the patient's condition, while also keeping a keen eye on the position of the ET tube by using continuous waveform capnography.

What Points Out the Need for ET Intubation?

ET intubation becomes necessary:

o In situations when there's a cardiac arrest or the protection of airway is needed and performing bag-mask ventilation is impossible or ineffective.

o In responsive patients that are experiencing respiratory symptoms or distress.

o Patients unable to protect their airway, either because of coma, areflexia, cardiac arrest, or other reasons

These are additional information and cautions health workers should pay attention to when using ET intubation.

• In cases where monitoring of the ET tube is inadequate, or untrained and inexperienced performs ET intubation on a client, fatal complications are unacceptably high.

• Out-of-hospital ET intubation records has shown that attempting to place ET tube intubation in the patient without the appropriate setting has led to complications and increased risk of dislodgment.

• It is possible for health workers to reduce the interruption time between chest compressions by inserting the laryngoscope blade while the tube is already at hand when compressions are paused. Interrupt compressions only to visualize the vocal cords and insert the tube; this is ideally less than 10 seconds. Resume chest compressions immediately after passing the tube between the vocal cords. Verify the tube's placement. If the initial intubation attempt is unsuccessful, healthcare providers may make a second attempt, but they should consider using a supraglottic airway.

Techniques Involved in Using ET Tube in Ventilating During Chest Compression

While performing ET intubation with patients with cardiac arrest, the following must be provided:

Volume

— This volume ought to make visible chest rise to occur.

— While practicing this skill, one should understand what such volume feels like when squeezing the ventilation bag.

— Ensure to provide slightly more volume for patients who are very obese.

Rate

This means you would have to provide about 1 breath every 6 seconds when administering ventilation during CPR or respiratory arrest.

Compression-Ventilation Cycles

Immediately an advance airway management device is in place, the health worker should provide both continuous compressions and asynchronous ventilations once every 6 seconds. The health worker should ensure to switch compressors every 2 minutes.

In other words, whenever any advanced airway management is in place, the patient should be ventilated, especially during cardiac arrest, once every 6 seconds, while for patients in respiratory arrest, once every 5 to 6 seconds.

Some patients that suffer from increased resistance to exhalation, such as severe obstructive lung disease or asthma, have tendencies to have air trapped inside them. Air trapping could lead to positive end-expiratory pressure effect that could considerably lower blood-pressure. For such patients, a slower ventilation rates which would allow complete exhalation should be used; while in cases of hypovolemia, ensure to restore intravascular volume.

Trauma That May Be Experienced by Patients as an Effect of ET Tube Usage

- Brain damage, or in severe cases, death

- This occurs if the ET tube is inserted to a patient's esophagus. This would mean that the patient would receive no oxygen unless he/she is still breathing spontaneously. If esophageal intubation is not quickly recognized, the patient could suffer acute and permanent brain damage, and could die as well.

- Lacerated lips or tongues which could be a result of a forceful pressure of the laryngoscope blade against the tongue or cheek.

- Chipped teeth

- Lacerated Pharynx or trachea as a result of the insertion of the stylet of the ET tube

- Vocal cords injury

- Pharyngeal-esophageal perforation

- Vomiting and emitting of gastric contents into the lower airway.

Procedure and Cautions to Take to Insert ET Tube into The Bronchus

Insertion of the ET tube into the Bronchus is frequent complication in the ET tube procedure. Though, it's more common for insertion to be at the right bronchus, but left bronchus insertion is not unheard of either. When bronchus intubation is not recognized and corrected, it could lead to hypoxemia due to under inflation of the uninvolved lung or over inflation of the ventilated lung.

In order to recognize an ET intubation, listen to the chest for bilateral sounds. Additionally, look for equal expansion of both sides of the chest during ventilation. The use of waveform capnography is not effective to recognize any main bronchus intubation.

If, by any chance, you suspect that either the left or the right bronchus has the ET tube inserted in it, take the following actions:

— Ensure the tube cuff is deflated

— Withdraw the tube back 1cm to 2 cm

— Make sure the ET tube is properly placed through clinical assessment and device confirmation.

- Reinflate the tube cuff, then secure the ET tube in position.

- Cross-check the clinical signs of the patient, which includes chest expansion, breath sound, and evidence of oxygenation.

When the ET tube has passed through the vocal cords, and its position is verified by auscultation and correct chest expansion during positive-pressure ventilation. You should ensure that everything is in proper order by obtaining additional information of proper placement using continuous quantitative waveform capnography or a qualitative device like a colorimetric $PETCO_2$ detector or EDD.

After the stability of the patient has been ascertained, the ET tube position, and the assessment of the lung pathology, can be further optimized through X-ray. Despite the additional advantage that X-ray provides, sometimes it takes too long to be taken and used for confirming tracheal placement, the responsibility of recognizing the misplacement of the ET tube, if any falls on the clinical team.

The recording and securing of the depth of the tube as marked at the front teeth or gums comes next after inserting and ascertaining the correct placement of the ET tube. It is prudent to secure the tube with tape, or a commercial device, just in case the patient is moved around, and the ET tube is moved with the head flexion of the patient. Though while applying the tape, ensure it does not interfere with the compression of the front and sides of the neck, as this could lead to impairment of venous return from the brain.

Immediately after the ET tube has been placed or when the patient is moved, confirm its correct placement by assessing the first administered breath of the bag-mask device. The health worker should utilize both clinical assessment and device confirmation to verify the correct tube placement.

Despite all these precautions, there is no single confirmation techniques is completely reliable, especially when patients with cardiac arrest is concerned. The use of continuous waveform capnography in addition to clinical assessment is recommended as the most combined reliable method to adequately confirm the correct placement of the ET tube.

In cases where waveform capnography is not accessible, EDD or non-waveform PETCO2 monitor, in addition to clinical assessment can be used to correctly ascertain the confirmation of the correct ET tube placement.

Assessing the correct placement of ET tube through physical examination includes visualization of the bilateral chest expansion, and listening over the epigastrium, which means breath sounds should not be heard, and the lung fields bilaterally, which means breath sounds should be equal and adequate.

While the bag is squeeze, listen over the epigastrium, and observe the movement of the chest wall. If you hear the stomach gurgle and see no chest-wall expansion, then that means the esophagus has been intubated. Stop the ventilators immediately and remove the ET tube at once.

Then carry out these following options:

In situations when CPR is already in progress continue the chest compressions

You can either resume the bag-mask ventilation or consider another alternative device to manage the advanced airway.

Only attempt to intubate the patient again after the patient has been re-oxygenated; about 30 seconds of 100% pure bag-mask ventilation is required.

In cases when, after intubation, the chest walls of the patient rises normally and stomach gurgling is not heard, listen to the lung fields with 5-point auscultation over the left/right anterior of the lung fields, over the stomach and left/right of the mid-axillary lung fields. Ensure the location of the breath sound is properly recorded in the patient's record file. If any doubt exists as to the exact location of the breathing sound, stop tube ventilations, then use the laryngoscope to check if the tube is actually going through the vocal cords.

If doubts still exist after this, remove the tube completely, and administer bag-mask ventilation to till the tube can be re-inserted.

If there's no doubt and the tube still seem to be correctly placed, cross-check the tube mark, usually at the front teeth. The tube mark would have been previously noted after inserting the tube 1cm to 2 cm into the vocal cord.

It is ideal to secure the tube, either with commercial device made for that purpose. Do ensure that in securing the tube, you avoid compressions of the front and sides of the neck as that could be fatal.

There are some commercial devices designed to serve as bite-block also. But if the commercial device used does not serve this purpose, insert a bite-block to prevent the patient from biting down and disrupting the away.

It is recommended to get confirmation by both clinical assessment and a device in a view to ensure the correct placement of the ET Tube. In order to increase the efficiency of the ET tube and decrease the interruption time of chest compressions, it is also recommended that the device is attached to the bag before it is joined to the tube.

Numerous research and assessment has shown that out-of-hospital ET tube intubation are much more difficult due to poor setting, and this has increased the chances of misplacement or displacement which could lead to fatal complications. Proper training and monitoring, frequent supervision and clinical experience, and process of quality improvement are all important part of a successful ET intubation, and these are absent in ET tube intubation.

In addition to physical assessment method, continuous waveform capnography is another reliable method of checking and monitoring the correct placement of an ET tube. The health workers should observe a continuous capnography waveform with ventilation in order to confirm and monitor the intubation of ET tube placement out of hospital, while in the transport vehicle, while arriving at the hospital, and while/after transferring the patient in order to prevent, and reduce to the barest minimum, any form of unrecognized tube misplacement and displacement which could lead to fatal complications. Using continuous waveform capnography to ascertain the correct placement of the ET tube has shown high sensitivity and specify in correctly recognizing a correct ET tube placement or otherwise.

Although the use of capnography to ascertain and supervise the placement of supraglottic airways has not been effectively researched, effective ventilation of a patient through a supraglottic airway device should result in a capnography waveform during CPR and after return of spontaneous circulation (ROSC).

Capnometry Functions

What a Capnometry does is to show a single quantitative read-out of the carbon dioxide (CO_2) concentration at a single point in time. It provides a continuous display of the CO_2 level as it differs throughout the cycle of ventilation.

The results of this display can help to confirm the success of an ET tube insertion within seconds of insertion. They can also alarm health workers if the patient is deteriorating due to ET tube misplacement or displacement, or probably declining clinical status. ET tube displacement has grown in frequency; especially in patients who are being transported to a hospital.

Commercial devices used in securing ET tubes can react to CO2 exhaled from the lungs by changing colors; different devices react differently i.e., change to different colors. If this simple method is used by an experienced health worker, it can be an effective alternative for recognizing correct or incorrect tube placement if the continuous waveform capnography is not available. Note that there is no supported evidence to show that these commercial devices are accurate in their predictions.

Also note that, using carbon dioxide detection cannot ensure proper depth of ET tube insertion, also the ET tube should only secure when proper placement has been ascertained. There's also the risk of identify how the commercial device would react since different device change to different colors.

EDD Functions

EDD also known as *Esophageal Detector Devices* is used to find the location of the distal end of the ET tube by using simple anatomical principles. It does not rely on blood flow, unlike the end-tidal CO_2 detector. The EDD is best used before any breath is given to the patient and health worker should compress the bulb-style EDD completely before attaching it to the ET tube. If, after the bulb has been released, it lies on the esophagus, the bulb should be re-inflated. This re-inflation process would produce a vacuum which would pull the esophageal mucosa against the tip of the tube. This would result in slow, or in some cases, no re-expansion of the bulb.

The syringe-style EDDs operate differently. With this type of EDD, the vacuum occurs when the rescuer pulls back on the syringe plunger. If the ET tube is placed in the esophagus, the health worker would be unable to pull back on the trigger; and if the rube lies on the trachea, the vacuum will allow smooth re-expansion of the bulb or aspiration of the syringe.

In situations where waveform capnography is not within reach, an EDD, used by an experienced operator, is also an effective alternative to either confirm or correct ET tube placement.

However, there are some results by some observation studies and small controlled trials that has reported a low false-positive rate for confirming tracheal placement, though there is no evidence to support the fact that an EDD is precise or practical for the purpose of continued monitoring of ET tube placement.

Note that in patients with from morbid obesity, late pregnancy or status asthmaticus, the EDD may likely yield misleading results.

CARDIAC ARREST RHYTHMS AND CONDITIONS

Patients in cardiac arrest have, as their ECG rhythms or conditions, ventricular fibrillation (VF) pulseless ventricular tachycardia (VT), asystole, pulseless electrical activity (PEA), which presents with a variety of rhythms.

These ECG rhythms are shown and discussed in the categories below:

- Ventricular fibrillation
- Pulseless electrical activity
- Asystole
- Atrial fibrillation and atrial flutter
- Accessory-Mediated SVT e.tc

Ventricular Fibrillation

The ventricles of a healthy heart comprise of areas of normal myocardium that's constantly alternating with areas of ischemic. Injured or infected Myocardium would lead to a chaotic asynchronous pattern of ventricular depolarization and repolarization. Without an organized depolarization system, the ventricles would not be able to contract as unit. In other words, they would produce no cardiac output, and the heart would only beat but not pump blood.

Standard for Evaluation in Accordance with ECG

- **Amplitude:** This is measured from peak deflection to trough deflection. It is often used specifically to describe VF as fine, which is peak to trough 2 to <5 mm, medium (or moderate), which is 5 to < 10 mm, coarse, which is 10 to <15 mm, or very coarse, which is >15.

- **Rate/QRS complex:** Inability to ascertain; undetectable P, QRS, or T waves; baseline undulation is usually between 150 and 500 per minute.

- **Rhythm:** Indeterminate; pattern of sharp up deflection, also known as peak deflection, and down deflection, also known as trough deflection.

Physical Effects

The Pulse would disappear with immediate introduction of VF. In some cases, the pulse may disappear before the introduction of VF if a common precursor to VF, which is Rapid VT, is developed before the VF.

- Collapse or Unresponsiveness

- Apnea; or in some cases, agony gasps

- Sudden death

- Common Etiologies

- Untreated stable or unstable VT

- Premature ventricular complexes (PVCs) with R-On-T sausage.

- ACS that could very lead to ischemic areas of myocardium

- Primary (minor) or Secondary (critical) QT prolongation

- Electrolyte, Multiple drug, or acid-base abnormalities that prolong the relative refractory period

- Electrocution, hypoxia; and many others

  The following are the ECG Criteria for VF:

- Rhythm: There is no discernible regular rhythmic pattern. The electrical waveforms may also vary in size or shape while the pattern is completely disorganized.

- QRS Complexes: It is impossible to recognize a normal-looking QRS complex. In other words, it is impossible to see a regular negative-positive-negative pattern (Q-R-S).

- Rate: The rates of electrical deflections are virtually uncountable. They are very fast, way too disorganized to be countable.

In relation to electrophysiology, prognosis and the likely clinical responses while attempting to defibrillate adrenergic agents or antiarrhythmics, it may be difficult to discern between the rhythm pattern of VF and Asystole.

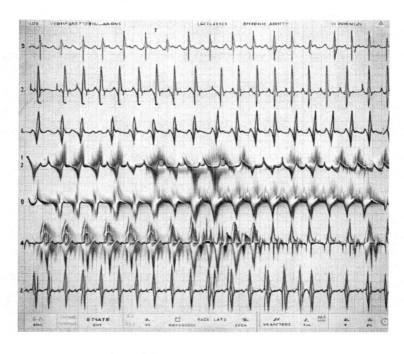

Rhythm Strip 1. Ventricular Fibrillation

Pulseless Electrical Activity

Sometimes, cardiac conduction impulses may occur in an organized pattern but unable to produce myocardial contraction. This condition was formerly called electromechanical dissociation. It is usually caused by insufficient ventricular filling during diastole or ineffective contractions.

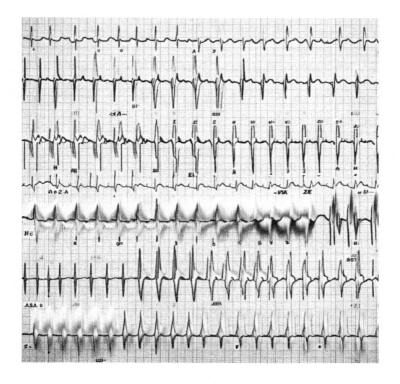

Rhythm Strip 2. Pulseless electrical activity

Standard for Evaluation in Accordance with ECG

- The Rhythm displays organized electrical activity, and not VF or pulseless VT.

- It is usually not as organized as a normal sinus rhythm

- It can be narrow, which is QRS <0.12 second, or wide, which is QRS ≥0.12 second, fast, which is > 100 beats per minute, or slow, which is <60 beats per minute.

- While fast rate heart and narrow QRS are caused by non-cardiac etiology, slow heart rate and wide QRS are mostly caused by cardiac etiology.

Physical Effects

- Collapse or Unresponsiveness

- Apnea; or in some cases, agony gasps

- Palpitation is unable to detect any pulse; very low systolic blood pressure could still be detectable in such cases

Common Etiologies

- Hypoxia

- Hypothermia

- Cardiac Tamponade

- Coronary Thrombosis (ACS)

- Hypo/hyperkalemia

- Tension Pneumothorax

- Hypovolemia

- Hydrogen ion, also called Acidosis

- Pulmonary Thrombosis, also called Embolism

Asystole

Asystole commonly presents itself as a flat line while the defining criteria are virtually non-existent.

Standard for Evaluation of Asystole in Accordance with ECG

- **Rate:** There is no seen ventricular activity, also called P-wave asystole, which is only seen in atrial impulses present (P waves).

- **Rhythm:** There is no seen ventricular activity.

- **PR:** It cannot usually be determined. Occasionally, the P-wave is present and visible, but by general rule, the R-wave must always be absent.

- **QRS Complex:** The visible detections are inconsistent with a QRS Complex

Physical Results

- Collapse or Unresponsiveness

- Low blood pressure or no pulse

- Death

- Apnea; or in some cases, agony gasps

Common Etiologies

- Cardiac ischemia

- Huge electrical shock, which may be in form of electrocution, lighting strike etc.

- May represent "stunning" of the heart immediately after defibrillation (shock delivery that eliminates VF) before resumption of spontaneous rhythm

- No oxygen, apnea or asphyxiation could lead to acute respiratory failure or hypoxia.

- Death

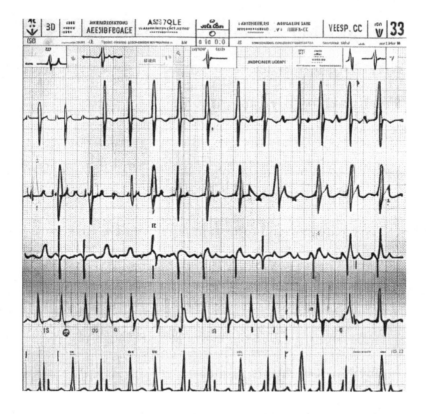

Rhythm Strip 3. Asystole

Recognizing Selected Non-Arrest ECG Rhythm and Super ventricular Tachyarrhythmias

- It is more like a physical response or signal than an actual arrhythmia or pathologic condition

- The conduction and formation of the impulse are normal

ECG Features and Defining Criteria of Selected Non-Arrest ECG Rhythm and Super ventricular Tachyarrhythmias:

- **Rate:** The rate is more than 100 beats per minute

- **Rhythm:** The rhythm is sinus

- **PR:** Normally about less than 0.20 seconds

- **P for every QRS complex**

- **QRS Complex:** The complex may be either normal or wide. It depends largely on the underlying abnormality

Physical Results

- There is no specific physical effect for the tachycardia.

- There could be presence of symptoms due to the cause of tachycardia. These symptoms include hypovolemia, fever, etc.

Common Etiologies

- Anemia

- Hyperthyroidism

- Fever

- Hypoxemia

- Normal Exercise

- Pain

- Anxiety due to Adrenergic stimulation

Atrial Fibrillation and Atrial Flutter

Atrial fibrillation makes the heartbeat at a faster rate beyond the range 60 to 100 times a patient heart is expected to beat per minute while the patient is at rest. While a rhythm disorder which causes the upper chambers of the heart to beat at a very fast rate is known as atrial flutter. The impulses of the Atrial are faster than the impulses of the Sinoatrial, also called SA nose, impulses.

- The impulses of the Atrial fibrillation take random multiple chaotic paths through the Atria

- For Atrial Flutter, the impulses take a circular course around the Atria, and setting up flutter waves in the process

Defining Criteria and ECG Features of Arial Fibrillation

- **Atrial Fibrillation Key:** The variation in both amplitude and interval from R-wave to R-wave is what is exactly known as Atrial fibrillation. The classic clinical axioms of the R-wave to R-wave is of an 'irregularly irregular rhythm'. This one is commonly reliable and can be observed in a multifocal atrial tachycardia (MAT).

- **Atrial Flutter Key:** The flutter waves of R-wave to R-wave are in a classical 'zigzag' pattern.

The two distinctions mentioned above are the only differences between atrial flutter and atrial fibrillation, all other features are actually the same.

Rate for Atrial Fibrillation

- The ventricular undulation responds in a wide-ranging manner and occur between 300 to 400 beats per minute.

- The rate of the undulation may be normal or slow depending on the abnormality of the atrioventricular (AV) nodal conduction, e.g., sick sinus syndrome

Rhythm: The rhythm of the undulation is irregular.

P Waves: The fibrillatory only creates chaotic waves with variable baseline.

PR: It cannot be measure

QRS: The QRS remains at less than 0.12 per second unless the QRS complex is disturbed by conduction defects through ventricles, flutter waves or fibrillation.

Rate for Atrial flutter

- The Atrial rate is about 220 to 250 beats per minute

- The Ventricular responses are either a function of AV node block or conduction of atrial impulses, though ventricular response is barely less than 150 to 180 due to the conduction limits of AV nodal.

Rhythm: The rhythm of the atrial flutter is regular; and the atrial rhythm is set to regular ratio e.g. 2:1 or 4:1

P Waves: Though there are no visible true P waves, the flutter waves occur in a classic "zigzag" pattern.

Physical Effects

- Both the Atrial flutter and atrial fibrillation can be asymptomatic.

- Absence of 'Atrial Kick' could lead to both decreased coronary perfusion and reduced cardiac output

- Irregular rhythm is frequently confused for palpitations

- The rate at which the ventricular responds to atrial fibrillation waves is mostly a function of signs and symptoms. For example, symptoms like dyspnea on exertion, shortness of breath, and. in some cases, acute pulmonary edema are a tell-tale sign of atrial fibrillation with rapid ventricular response.

Common Etiologies

- Sepsis

- Hyperthyroidism

- Hypertension

- Hypoxia

- Mitral or tricuspid valve disease

- Acute coronary syndrome, or in some cases, coronary artery disease or congestive heart failure

- Drug-induced: digoxin or quinidine.

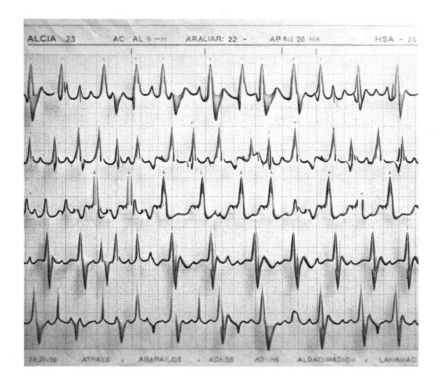

Rhythm Strip 4. Atrial flutter

93

Accessory-Mediated SVT

This may include AV reentry tachycardia or AV nodal reentrant tachycardia. The reentry phenomenon includes repeated impulses recycle in the AV node due an abnormal rhythm circuit which allows the depolarization wave to travel in a circle. Normally, the depolarization waves would travel forward, that is in an ante-grade movement, through the abnormal pathway. It would then come back around, which is retrograde, through the normal conduction tissue.

Standard for Evaluation of Accessory-Mediated SVT in Accordance to ECG

The key is the usual narrow-complex tachycardia that occurs without warning, P waves or cessation. Note that, some experts require the capture of the abrupt onset or cessation on a monitor strip to determine the diagnosis of SVT re-entry.

Rate: The rate of this SVT goes above the upper limit of a Sinus tachycardia at rest, which is less than 220 beats per minute. Though it could often go up to 250 beats per minute, it rarely goes below 150 beats per minute.

Rhythm: The rhythm is regular

P waves: The P waves are rarely seen. This is because rapid rate often causes P Wave to be difficult to recognize because the origin id low in the atrium or hidden in preceding T waves.

QRS complex: The QRS complex are normal and narrow.

Physical Results of Accessory-Mediated SVT

- The immediate palpitations patients feel makes them anxious and uncomfortable

- The exercises are of low tolerance with very high rates

- The symptoms associated with unstable tachycardia may occur

Common Etiologies

- Patients suffering from coronary artery disease, chronic obstructive pulmonary disease, and congestive heart failure often experience increased in SVT frequency.

- Many SVT patients experience accessory conduction pathway.

- Otherwise seen in healthy people, factors such as caffeine, hypoxia, cigarettes, stress, anxiety, sleep deprivation, numerous medications can provoke the reentry of SVT

Ventricular Tachyarrhythmias Recognition Monomorphic VT

- Areas with ventricular injury, or ischemia, often experience reduced conduction of impulse

- These areas also double as the source of ectopic impulses, also called irritable foci.

- The impulse conduction can be forced to take a circular course due to the areas of injury. This often leads to re-entry phenomenon and rapid repetitive depolarization.

Standard for Evaluation of Ventricular Tachyarrhythmias Recognition Monomorphic VT in Accordance to ECG

- **Key:** The same morphology is noticed in every QRS Complex. Note that, there are more consecutive PVCs indicated in VT; and the VT with less than 30 seconds duration is known as non-sustained VT, while VT of more than 30 seconds is known as Sustained VT

- **Rate:** Typically, the ventricular rate is 120 to 250 beats per minute, but it could reach less than 100 beats per minute.

- **Rhythm:** The ventricular rhythm is regular, and AV dissociated

- **PR:** The PR is absent

- **P Waves:** Though the P waves are barely seen, they're present. A VT is a form of AV dissociation, a defining characteristic for wide-complex tachycardias of ventricular origin versus supraventricular tachycardias with aberrant conduction

- **QRS Complex:** The QRS Complex is wide and quite strange, in that the PVC-like complexes are ≥ 0.12 second, with large T wave of opposite polarity from QRS.

- **Fusion beats:** There are occasional cases where a conducted P wave is mistakenly captured. This would result in a QRS hybrid complex that is part normal and part ventricular

- **Non-sustained VT:** This type of VT barely lasts less than 30 seconds, and do not require intervention.

Physical Effects:

- With Monomorphic VT, symptoms that indicate decreased cardiac output often develop. These symptoms include orthostasis, hypotension, syncope, exercise limitations, etc.

- Sustained VT that are left untreated will deteriorate to unstable Vt, and most times, into VF.

- Despite the widespread belief that sustained VT always produces symptoms, Monomorphic VT can also be asymptomatic.

Common Etiologies

- PVCs that occur during relative refractory period of cardiac cycle is often called R-on-T phenomenon

- Drug-induced prolonged QT interval, such as, tricyclic antidepressants, procainamide, sotalol, amiodarone, butizide, dovetailed, some antipsychotics, digoxin, some long-acting antihistamines and some certain antibiotics.

- Reduced ejection fraction which is commonly caused by systolic heart failure

- An acute ischemic situation caused by areas of ventricular irritability, and leading to PVCs

Polymorphic VT

- Areas with Ventricular injury, infarct, or ischemia causes impulse condition to slow down

- These affected areas also double as the origin of ectopic impulses, also called Irritable foci.

- Irritable Foci are polymorphic, in that, they appear in multiple areas of the affected ventricles

- The impulse conduction can be forced to take a circular course due to the areas of injury. This often leads to re-entry phenomenon and rapid repetitive depolarization.

Standard for Evaluation of Polymorphic VT in Accordance with ECG

- **Key**: The variations are marked and are inconsistent, as seen in QRS complexes

- **Rate:** The rate at which the ventricular beats is greater than 100 beats per minute, which, typically, is 120 to 250 beats per minute.

- **Rhythm:** The rhythm of the ventricular is either regular or irregular, and there is no presence of atrial activity

- **PR:** Non-existent

- **P-Waves:** The P waves are rarely seen but they are present, while VT is a form or AV dissociation.

- **QRS Complex:** The variations are marked and are inconsistent, as seen in QRS complexes

Physical Effect

- Before the pulseless arrest, the symptoms of reduced cardiac output are already present. These symptoms include, orthostasis, hypotension, poor perfusion, syncope, etc.

- Untreated, it will rapidly deteriorate to either pulseless VT or VF.

Common Etiologies

- Hereditary long QT interval syndromes

- PVCs that occur during relative refractory period of cardiac cycle is often called R-on-T phenomenon

- Drug-induced prolonged QT interval, such as, tricyclic antidepressants, procainamide, sotalol, amiodarone, ibutilide, dofetilide, some antipsychotics, digoxin, some long-acting antihistamines and some certain antibiotics.

- Reduced ejection fraction which is commonly caused by systolic heart failure

- An acute ischemic situation caused by areas of ventricular irritability, and leading to PVCs

Torsades De Pointes

Torsades De Pointes is a potentially fatal situation in which the heart's lower chambers don't beat in accordance to the heart's upper chamber. torsades come with this specific pathophysiology.

The QT interval, which is the baseline ECG, is very long and leads to a spike in the relative refractory period, also called vulnerable period of the cardiac cycle. This spike increases the probability that an irritable focus, PVC, will occur on the T-wave. This phenomenon is called the R-On-T phenomenon which often induces VT.

Standard for Evaluation of Torsades De Pointes in Accordance with ECG

- **Key:** A 'spindle-node' shape is displayed on the QRS complexes. This occurs when the increased VT amplitude caused a reduction in the regular pattern, thereby creating the Spindle. The initial deflection at the start of one spindle (e.g., negative) will be followed by complexes of opposite (e.g., positive) polarity or deflection at the start of the next spindle, creating the node.

- **Atrial Rate:** The atria rate cannot be ascertained

- **Ventricular Rate:** The Ventricular rate complexes beat around 150 to 250 per minute.

- **Rhythm:** The ventricular rhythm is irregular

- **PR:** Non-existent

- **QRS complexes:** The QRS complex is displayed in a classic spindle node pattern

Physical Effects

- The stable torsades, which is a sustained torsades, is quite uncommon

- There is a possibility of a sudden deterioration to pulseless VT or VF

- There would be visible symptoms of decreased cardiac output, which includes; orthostasis, hypotension, syncope, signs of poor perfusion, etc.)

Common Etiologies

- Critical ischemic events

- Inherited forms of long QT syndrome

- It occurs frequently in cases that have patients with prolonged QT interval. Some major reasons are;

o They might be drug-induced. These drugs include tricyclic antidepressants, procainamide, sotalol, amiodarone, ibutilide, dofetilide, some antipsychotics, digoxin, some long-acting antihistamines, and some certain antibiotics.

o Alterations to the electrolyte and metabolism

Sinus Bradycardia Recognition

The impulse originated at the SA node is usually at a slow rate. This could be a physiologic sign, or physical sign, as seen in sinus tachycardia.

Standard for Evaluation in Accordance to ECG

Key: The regular QRS are followed by the regular P waves at the rate of less than 60 beats per minute. Although, there is usually a physical sign, an abnormal rhythm also occurs.

Rate: Usually, the rate is less than 60 beats per minute, but when symptomatic and/or bradycardia is the cause of symptoms, the rate is generally less than 50 beats per minute.

Rhythm: The Sinus rhythm is regular

PR: The PR is regular and is between 0.12 to 0.20 second

P-Waves: Both the size and shape are normal while every P wave is followed by a QRS complex and vice versa

QRS Complex: The QRS complex is narrow and less than 0.12 second, though often goes less than 0.11 second in cases where the of intraventricular conduction defect is absent.

Physical Effects Include

- The patient is usually asymptomatic when at rest

- The ECG result could either display severe ST-segment, T-wave deviation or ventricular arrhythmias.

104

- A slow consistent rate can, with increased activity and sinus node dysfunction, result to shortness of breath, easy tiredness, light-headedness or dizziness, syncope hypotension, diaphoresis, pulmonary congestion, and frank pulmonary edema.

Common Etiologies

- Vomiting, Valsalva maneuver, rectal stimuli, and other vasovagal occurrences cans cause inadvertent pressure on carotid Sinus, otherwise called Shaver's Syncope.

- Adverse drug effects

- Acute coronary syndromes that affect circulation to SA node which is the right coronary artery, and, most often, affect the inferior acute myocardial infarctions (AMIs)

AV Block Recognition

The impulse conduction is either slowed or partially blocked at the AV node for a fixed interval. This may be a sign of either another problem or basically an abnormality in conduction

Standard for Evaluation in Accordance with ECG

- **Key:** The PR interval is usually >0.20 second

105

- **Rate:** First-degree AV blocks, as well as Sinus brachy cardia, Sinus tachycardia, and normal Sinus mechanism are seen.

- **Rhythm:** The rhythm of both the sinus atria and ventricles are regular

- **PR:** The PR is prolonged and fixed at less than 0.20 second

- **P Waves:** Both the size and shape are normal while every P wave is followed by a QRS complex and vice versa

- **QRS Complex:** The QRS complex is narrow and less than 0.12 second where the of intraventricular conduction defect is absent.

Physical Effect

It is usually asymptomatic.

Common Etiologies

- Any event or condition that stimulates the parasympathetic nervous system such as vomiting.

- The AMI usually affects the AV node circulation of the coronary artery, and most commonly the inferior AMI

- The reason for many first-degree AV blocks is due to drugs, such as non-dihydropyridine calcium channel blockers, and digoxin

Type One Second Degree Av Block

The AV node is the site of the Pathology which supplies blood from the branches of the right coronary artery, dominating the right circulation. The AV node steadily slows the conduction of the impulse, thereby causing increasing PR interval until one sinus impulse is completely blocked and the QRS complex cannot follow.

Standard for Evaluation in Accordance with ECG

- **Key:** The PR interval of one P Wave till its followed by QRS is progressive lengthening.

- **Rate:** The atrial rate is just a little bit faster than ventricular rate mainly because of reduced conduction, though it's still normally within normal range.

- **Rhythm:** Due to dropped beats, both Atrial and Ventricular complexes have irregular timing. It often shows the regular P waves marching through irregular QRS

- **PR:** The progressive lengthening of the PR interval normally happens from cycle to cycle.

- **P Waves:** Both size and shape remain normal; and, seldom, the P Wave is not followed by the QRS complex

- **QRS Complex:** It is commonly less than 0.12 second, but sometimes QRS periodically drop.

Physical Effect

- Because of bradycardia, most symptoms are often asymptomatic. Signs and Symptoms may include Chest pain, shortness of breath, decreased level of consciousness, hypotension, shock, pulmonary congestion, congestive heart failure, angina

Common Etiologies

- The right coronary artery is commonly plagued with severe coronary syndrome

- Situations that provoke the parasympathetic nervous system into action

- AV nodal blocking agents, such as beta-blockers, non-dihydropyridine calcium channel blockers, digoxin

Type 2 Second Degree Av Block

Mostly, the site is located below the AV, also called the intranodal, at either the HIS, also called infrequent, or bundle branches. The impulse conduction normally passes through the node, hence there is no prior PR prolongation or first-degree block.

Standard for Evaluation in Accordance with ECG

- **Atrial Rate:** This usually 60 to 100 beats per minute.

- **Ventricular Rate:** Due to blocked impulses, the ventricular rate is slower than atrial rate

- **Rhythm:** While atrial rhythm is regular, ventricular rhythm is irregular, due to blocked impulses. The ventricular regular is regular if there is consistent 2:1 or 3:1 block.

- **PR:** The PR is fixed and constant while there is no progressive prolongation; a major distinguishing characteristic between Type 1 and Type 2 second degree AV block.

- **P Waves:** The size is normal both size and shape. The P waves impulse conduction are absent hence not able to be followed by QRS complex

- **QRS Complex:** The QRS Complex could either be narrow and less 0.12 seconds, indicating that the high block is relative to AV node or wide, ≥0.12 second, indicating that the low block is relative to AV node.

Physical Effects

- Because of bradycardia, most signs and symptoms may include Chest pain, shortness of breath, decreased level of consciousness, hypotension, shock, pulmonary congestion, congestive heart failure, angina

Common Etiologies

- The right coronary artery is commonly plagued with severe coronary syndrome

Third Degree Av Block and Av Dissociation

There is a complete block of cardiac conduction system between the Atria and the Ventricles, so that no impulses can pass between them, neither ante-grade retrograde. This complete block can happen at several different anatomic areas such as Bundle of HIS, Bundle branches, both low nodal or infranodal, or the high, supra or junctional AV nodal block.

Standard for Evaluation in Accordance to ECG

- **Key:** The complete block makes both the atria and the ventricular to depolarize independently with AV dissociation, i.e. with no relationship between the both of them.

- **Atrial rate:** The rate is commonly between 60 to 100 beats per minute while the impulse rate of the atrial is independent from the slower ventricular rate.

- **Ventricular rate**: The rate at which the ventricular beats escape the rise determines the ventricular rate. If the ventricular escape rate is slower than atrial rate than that would equal third-degree AV block at the rate of 20 to 40 beats per minute, but if the ventricular escape rate is faster than atrial rate then that would equal AV dissociation at the rate of 40 to 55 beats per minute.

- **Rhythm:** The atrial and ventricular rates are independent but have a regular rhythm

- **PR:** There is no relationship between the P wave and the R wave

- **P waves:** Both the size and shape are normal.

- **QRS Complex**: The QRS Complex could either be narrow and less 0.12 seconds, indicating that the high block is relative to AV node or wide, ≥ 0.12 second, indicating that the low block is relative to AV node.

Physical Effects

- Because of bradycardia, most signs and symptoms may include Chest pain, shortness of breath, decreased level of consciousness, hypotension, shock, pulmonary congestion, congestive heart failure, angina

Common Etiologies

- The right coronary artery is commonly plagued with severe coronary syndrome

- This coronary syndrome also affects the LAD (Left Anterior Descending) artery and branches supplies the bundle branches to the interventricular septum

Defibrillation

Health workers that provide ACLS will normally utilize a manual defibrillator to shock a patient into VF or, in some cases, pulseless VT. In some situations, only an AED, Automated External Defibrillator, is available for use. The only times that AEDs are to be used on a patient are when clinical findings:

- Finds no response in the patient

- Report an absent or abnormal breathing in the patient, i.e., no breathing, or in some cases, only gasping

- Find no pulse in the patient

The Patient may display agonal gasps in the first few minutes, or immediately, of a sudden cardiac arrest. This gasp may not suffice for the patient to breath well. A non-responsive cardiac arrest patient with agonal gasping may have no pulse.

Different AEDs are used in different clinical settings. Health worker must be very familiar with the AED used in their clinical setting and ensure that it is always ready to be used. Ensure to troubleshoot the device in accordance with the manufacturer's checklist while performing daily maintenance checks. These daily checks serve to ensure that the AED is ever ready to use, and also as an effective review step in any operation.

After the AED is in place, place it gently but firmly on the patient's side, right next to the operator. This position allows the operator to easily use the AED while easily controlling the electrode pads. It also enables a second operator to perform CPR from the opposite of the patient without interrupting the AED operation

AEDs come in different model with little variations between them. Despite these minor variations, they all operate in essentially the same way. Below are universal steps to follow in order to properly operate an AED.

Step 1: Open the carrying case, and power on the AED is need be, though some models would power on immediately the lid or case is open. Ensure to follow the AED prompts to guide you to the next steps.

Step 2: Latch the AED pads to the patient's bare chest. For patients that are 8 years or older, use adult pads and/or adult system. Follow these steps:

• Peel the backing away from the AED pads.

• Attach the adhesive AED pads to the patient's bare chest

- Though some AEDS are already pre-connected to the devices, ensure to hook the AED connecting cables to the AED device

Step 3: After 'clearing' the patient, let the AED analyze the rhythm of the patient. Do this by:

- Clear the victim during analysis when the AED prompts you to do so. Ensure that no one is touching the patient, not even the second operator giving breaths to the patients.

- While some AED would prompt you to push a button to allow the AED to analyze the heart rhythm, some AEDs would do it automatically. Analyzing may take a few seconds, depending on the model, and the AED informs you if a shock is needed.

Step 4: If the AED suggests a shock on the patient, it will inform you to clear the victim and then deliver a shock. To do this:

- Clear the patient before administering the shock but ensure no one is touching the patient.

- Articulate clearly and loudly a clearing the patient message, such as 'Clear'

- Double check to ensure no one is touching the patient, then shock the patient.

- The patient's muscles would suddenly contract due to the shock.

Step 5: If there's no need for shock or after shock delivery, immediately resume CPR, starting with chest compressions.

Step 6: After about 2 minutes of 5 cycles of CPR, the AED will prompt you to re-do steps 3 and 4.

Ensure to immediately resume high-quality CPR that starts with chest compressions, after:

- A shock is delivered; or

- The AED prompts 'no shock advised'

After about 5 cycles or 2 minutes of high-quality CPR, the AED will prompt you to repeat steps 3 and 4. Continue until advanced life support providers take over or the patient begins to breathe, move, or otherwise react.

There are only four conventional, and acceptable, AED electrode pad positions. They are:

- Anterolateral

- Anteroposterior

- Anterior–left infrascapular

- Anterior–right infrascapular

  These 4 pad placement positions are equally effective and used for defibrillation. Though, the anterolateral is the easiest and default placement, health workers may as very well consider alternative pad positions based on the patient's unique characteristics.

AED Analysis

Research made into causes of AED failure shows that most failures are caused by operator effects rather than by AED defects. Though Operator error would have a low probability of happening if the operator is experienced with the use of AED, had had recent trainings or practice with the AED, and is using a well-maintained AED.

In situations where AED does not immediately analyze the heart rhythm of the patient, do the following:

- Resume high-quality chest compressions and ventilations

- Check all the connecting cables between the AED and the patient to make sure they're all secured

Ensure that Chest compressions are not delayed or interrupted while troubleshooting the AED.

Should CPR or Shock Be First Attempted to an Adult Cardiac Arrest Patient?

The answer is that health workers that treat cardiac arrests in hospitals should provide immediate CPR until the AED or fibrillator is available and ready for use. In other words, use the AED as soon as it's available for use. Though, the advantage that defibrillation has over CPR is yet to be fully understood, EMS medical directors may consider utilizing a protocols that enables EMS responders to provide CPR to a patient while preparing the patient for AED or defibrillator. In other words, though AED should take more importance on a patient with cardiac arrest over CPR, CPR can be performed on the patient while the AED is getting ready.

When it comes to in-hospital patients suddenly going into cardiac arrest, Defibrillation should come before CPR. However, in monitored patients, the time from VF to defibrillation should be under 3 minutes. If there are 2 or more health worker present, one of them should begin CPR on the patient, while the other health worker activates the emergency response system and prepare the defibrillator.

When AED is Needed

There are some peculiar situations that would warrant an operator to take extra precaution on placing the electrode pads while using an AED. Some of them are:

Hairy Chest.

Placing the AED pads on patients with hairy chest could mean that the pads may stick to the hair on the skin and not directly applied to the chest. If this happens, the AED will not properly analyze the heart rhythm of the patient and the ED would give a 'check electrode pad' warning message. When this happens, you should do the following while minimizing the interruptions in chest compressions.

Step 1: Press down firmly on each pad, if the pads stick to the hair and not to the skin.

Step 2: If the AED keeps flashing the 'check the pads' warning message, quickly pull off the pads as this will remove much of the hair.

Step 3: If too much hair remains in the spot where you'll place the pads, shave the area with the razor made available in the AED carrying case, or other razor, if not available.

Step 4: Put on a new set of pads and follow the voice prompts of the AED.

Water.

Be careful not to use and ED in water. Using AED on a patient that has water on their chest would conduct the electricity across the skin of the chest, thereby preventing an adequate shock dose to be delivered to the heart.

In situations where the patient is inside the water, pull the patient out of the water and clean the chest areas. If the patient is lying on ice, snow or in a small puddle, immediately apply the AED

Implanted Pacemaker.

Patients that are extremely vulnerable to sudden cardiac arrest usually have defibrillators/pacemakers implanted in them to automatically deliver shocks directly to the heart muscle in case a life-threatening arrhythmia is discovered. These devices can be easily recognized since they create a hard lump under the skin of the upper chest or abdomen. The size of these lumps could range from the size of a silver dollar bill or half deck cards, and is usually accompanied with a small overlying scar. Although a pacemaker is not a contraindication to use an AED, avoid placing the AED electrode pads directly over the device as they may interfere with each other. If an implanted defibrillator or pacemaker is detected under the skin of the patient, then take the following steps:

- If it's possible, avoid placing the AED electrode pad directly over the implanted device, but rather on either side of the device

- Take the usual steps for operating an AEDs

Transdermal Medication Patches.

Avoid placing the AED electrode directly on top of a medication patch, such as a patch of nitroglycerin, nicotine, pain medication, hormone replacement therapy, or antihypertensive medication. The medication patch may transfer the energy of the electrode pad to the heart, block it completely or cause small burns to the skin. To avoid causing these complications, remove the patch completely and wipe it completely clean before applying the AED on the patient. Do not delay the shock delivery and try to minimize interruptions in chest compressions.

Defibrillation and Safety

Use of Manual Defibrillator

Performing a rhythm check, as indicated by the ACLS Cardiac Arrest Algorithm, is an important part of using a manual defibrillator or monitor. A rhythm check can be done by latching the adhesive defibrillator electrode pads or placing the defibrillator paddles on the chest, using gel or an appropriate conduction surface, in order to lessen transthoracic impedance. It can also be performed by using a paddle quick look feature.

Adhesive electrode pads are as effective as paddles and gel pads/paste, and it also has the advantage of being able to place it before cardiac arrest occur in order to properly monitor and promptly deliver shock when necessary; it used routine used and favored by health workers instead of the standard paddles.

Both handheld paddles and self-adhesive pads of about 8 to 12 cm in diameter are advised for adult defibrillation. Though it's worthy of note that electrodes with 12 cm diameter have a higher defibrillation success rate while smaller electrodes of about 4.3 cm may be harmful and could cause myocardial necrosis. For handheld paddles and/or gel pads, ensure that the paddle is in full contact with the skin. Although smaller pads have been effective in VF for a short duration, the smallest pediatric pads can result in unacceptably high transthoracic impedance in larger children.

When patients receive early defibrillation, they can survive sudden cardiac arrests. VF is a common initial rhythm in out-of-hospital patients with sudden cardiac arrest that can be treated with defibrillation. The probability of a defibrillation being successful reduces with time, and VF can deteriorate to asystole within 10 to 15 minutes. To prevent this, ensure delay to delivering shock and chest compressions is minimized either adhesive electrode pads or paddles are being used. Approximately 20 to 30 seconds interval is the limit for interruption between chest compressions and shock delivery, any more time could be fatal. Once the CPR is in progress, chest compressions must continue until the defibrillator electrode adhesive pads are attached to the chest and the manual defibrillator is ready to analyze the rhythm of the heart of the patient.

Survival rate of the patient decreases with 7% to 10% with every minute that passes between collapse and defibrillation if no CPR is provided. If CPR is provided by a by-stander, the survival rate of the patient between collapse and defibrillation increases, and triple for witnessed SCA at most intervals to defibrillation.

If any health worker witnesses an out-of-hospital sudden cardiac arrest and an AED is available on-site, the health worker should start CPR on the patient and use the AED as soon as possible. Healthcare providers who treat cardiac arrest in hospitals and other facilities with AEDs onsite should provide immediate CPR and should use the AED/defibrillator as soon as it becomes available.

Immediately a VF or a pulseless VT is detected, immediately deliver one shock using the energy levels give below:

- **Biphasic:** This is device specific. The first delivered dose is a carefully selected energy of 120J with a rectilinear biphasic waveform and a first dose selected energy of 120J to 200J with a biphasic truncated exponential waveform. If the recommended dosage by the manufacturer regarding the specific dose is specific dose shown to be effective for elimination of VF, defibrillation at the maximal dose may be considered.
- **Monophasic:** The first delivered dose is 360J. If the VF continues after the first, second and subsequent shocks of 360J should be given.

CPR, pushing hard and fast at a rate of 100 to 120 compressions per minute, must resume immediately a single shock had been delivered CPR interruption must be minimized and must allow full chest recoil after each compression.

It's important for the defibrillator operator to clearly announce that a shock is about to be delivered on the patient, and also perform a quick visual check to ensure that no one is in contact with the patient. This is to ensure the safety and success of the defibrillation process, either manual or automated. The purpose of the clear warning the operator makes before each shock is delivered it to ensure the safety of all by making sure no one is making contact with the patient, and also to ensure that no oxygen is flowing across the patient's chest or openly flowing across the electrode pads. The warning should be short and quick in order to minimize the interruption from the last compression to the shock delivery.

There are no exact words to be used, but it is important that everyone is warned about an imminent shock delivery and they should stand clear. All personnel must remove their hands from the patients, remove their hands from anything that's in contact with the patient; and this includes the health worker holding a ventilation bag to the patient, the bag must be disconnected from the patient.

Additionally, the health worker in charge of airway management and ventilation must make sure that oxygen is not openly flowing around the electrode pads, in some cases paddles, or across the patient's chest.

Modern AEDs and manual defibrillators commonly use biphasic waveforms. Health workers must dedicate time to learn how the defibrillator in their clinical setting works and its energy setting. Also remember that, regardless of the type of defibrillator or waveform, prompt an early defibrillation in the presence of shockable rhythm increases the probability of the patient's survival.

ACCESS FOR MEDICATIONS

Using Peripheral Veins for IV Access

Hands and arms are the most common sites health workers use for IV access. Other favored sites include, dorsum of the hands, the wrists, and the antecubital fossae, while the preferred IV location or drug administration during CPR is the antecubital vein.

A Summary of Its Description

The superficial radial vein, a thick vein, runs from the radial view of the wrist and joins the median cephalic vein to form the cephalic vein. Superficial veins located on the ulnar side of the forearm runs to the elbow to join the median basilic vein to form the basilic vein. The cephalic vein of the forearm bifurcates into a Y in the antecubital fossa, becoming the median cephalic (laterally) and the median basilic (medially).

Process Involved

The antecubital fossa is the vein with the largest surface veins in the arms. Patients in circulatory collapse or cardiac arrest are firstly accessed through these veins. Select a point between the junctions of 2 antecubital veins; the veins there are the most stable making venipuncture more successful.

In cases where peripheral access is not possible, central access via the femoral veins should be consulted. This is considered as it ensures that chest compressions and other resuscitation interventions should not be interrupted, and potential vascular injuries can be better controlled at this site.

The third option, if upper extremity and central line is not accessible, is the peripheral leg vein.

Once access to vascular access is gained, these important principles must be followed to ensure the success of administering IV therapy.

- Immediately after a patient with cardiac arrest has been stabilized, remove the emergently inserted cannula and replace it with a new sterilized one. Strict aseptic technique is compromised in most emergency venipunctures, where speed is essential. This compromise is particularly likely when emergency vascular access is established outside the hospital because personnel and equipment are limited.
- IV solutions are commonly packaged in a durable plastic bottles or bags. Shake the bag before use in order to identify possible punctures that may contaminate the contents.

- Drugs that might be absorbed by the tube or plastic bag, such as IV nitroglycerin, should be avoided. If these drugs must be administered without any special infusion system, then drug absorption rate must be considered especially when the drug is titrated.

- The ideal rate of infusion should be set to, at least, 10 mL/h to keep the IV line open.

- Patients with spontaneous circulations and require drug infections, but not IV volume infusion, should have saline lock catheter systems since it's particularly good for them.

- Most modern systems allow drug and flush infusions and can be used without needless injection site. This can prevent any complications that may arise from needles sticks.

- Ensure the arm with the IV access does not hang off the bed, and aligns with the heart level, or slightly above the heart. This enables easy delivery of fluids and medication to the central circulation.

- Drugs should be peripherally delivered with a bolus of, at least, 20 mL of IV flush solution into patients with cardiac arrest. This flush rate would ensure that fluids are promptly delivered to the central circulation. Elevate the extremity for 10 to 20 seconds to facilitate drug delivery to the central circulation.

- There are some complications common to all IV techniques. These complications include hematomas, cellulitis, thrombosis, infiltration, and phlebitis. Systemic complications include sepsis, pulmonary thromboembolism, air embolism, and catheter fragment embolism. Health workers should be wary of them.

Access to Bone Marrow Injection

Also known as Intraosseous (IO) access, serves as a fast, safe, and dependable path for drugs and blood administration, crystalloids, and colloids.

Type and Use of Needles

This technique requires a rigid needle, preferably one designed for IO or Jamshidi-type bone marrow needle. Previously, adults and older children have a higher bone density that made it difficult for smaller IO needles to penetrate the bone without bending. Thanks to technological development of IO cannula systems, drill-type devices, IO access in older children and adult is now easier to obtain.

Sites for Intraosseous Infusion

A lot of sites are suitable for IO infusions. For older children and adults, these sites include; the humeral head, proximal tibia, medial malleolus, sternum, distal radius, distal femur, and anterior-superior iliac spine.

Indications and Administration

IO route can safely deliver resuscitation drugs, fluids, and blood products to the patient. It can also serve as an infusion for Continuous catecholamine.

The onset of action and drug levels after IO infusion during CPR are comparable to those for vascular routes of administration, including central venous access. Pay heed to the following while providing drugs and fluids by the IO route.

Ensure all IO medications are flushed with normal saline in order to enable easy delivery into the central circulation.

Infusion pump, pressure bag or forceful manual pressures should be used to deliver viscous drugs and/or fluid with rapid volume in order to offset the resistance of the emissary veins.

131

Some individuals have voiced an opinion high pressure of blood might lead to hemolysis, but studies on animal have invalidated this opinion.

Contraindications

- Continuous attempt to establish access in the same bone
- Infection of the overlying tissues
- Crush or fractures that are near or proximal to the access site
- Medical conditions that make the bone fragile, e.g. osteogenesis imperfect

Complications That May Result from Intraosseous Infusion

Complications that could arise with the use of IO infusion include lower extremity compartment syndrome or severe extravasation of drugs, and osteomyelitis. Though less than 1% patients actually have complication after IO infusion, and careful technique had even helped to reduce the number of complications.

Equipment Required

- Tape
- Skin disinfectant
- Syringe
- Isotonic crystalloid fluid
- Intravenous tubing
- Gloves
- IO needle, of about 15 to gauge, or bone marrow needle.

Procedure

Using the tibial tuberosity as an example of an access site, the procedures to take in order to successfully establish a successful IO access is given below. Commercial kits such as drill-type IO devices, are currently available, and health providers should follow the manufacturer's steps provided with the kit.

Step 1: Always ensure you follow universal precautions, such as disinfecting the overlying skin and surrounding the area with a suitable agent, while attempting vascular access. Locate the tibial tuberosity which is just below the knee joint. The insertion site is that flat part of the tibia that's about 1 or 2 finger widths below and medial to this bony prominence.

Step 2: To prevent the needle from clogging with bone or tissue, the stylet should be left in place during insertion. While stabilizing the leg to enable insertion, remember not to lace your hand behind the leg.

Step 3: Insert the needle slightly perpendicular to the tibia. When going through other IO access sites, place the IO needle slightly away from the nearest join space to reduce the probability of injuring the epiphysis or joint; but ensure to always keep the needle perpendicular to the bone in order to avoid bending. Additionally, ensure you're twisting, and not pushing, the needle. A twisting motion coupled with a firm, but gentle pressure is ideal. In some cases, the IO needles come with thread, these threads must be turned clockwise and screwed into the bone.

Step 4: Keep inserting the needle through the cortical bone, until it enters the marrow space; a sudden release or resistance would be a sign that the needle has entered the marrow space. At this point, if the needle is properly placed it would stand without support.

Step 5: Go through the following procedures for this step:

• Remove the stylet and attach a syringe

• Though blood or bone marrow may not be aspirated in every case, it is usually a sign of proper placement. The blood may be sent to the lab for further studies.

• Infuse a small volume of saline and observe for swelling at the insertion site. Also check the extremity behind the insertion site in case the needle has penetrated into and through the posterior cortical bone. Fluid should easily infuse with saline injection from the syringe with no evidence of swelling at the site.

• If you observe infiltration or swelling near or at the injection site, it shows that the test injection has failed. When this happens, remove the needle and proceed the procedure on another bone. In cases where the cortex of the bone is penetrated, if another needle is placed in the same site, fluids and drugs will escape from the original hole and infiltrate the surrounding tissues which could cause critical injury.

Step 6: You can either place a tape over the flange of the needle to provide support for the needle, place gauze padding on both sides of the needle for additional support, in order to stabilize the needle.

Step 7: While connecting the IV tubing, tape the IV tubing to the skin in order to avoid displacing the needle by putting tension on the tubing.

Step 8: You can deliver volume resuscitation by:

- Use syringe bolus via a medication port in the IV tubing (3-way stopcock not needed).
- Using a stopcock attached to the extension tubing or by infusion or fluid under pressure.
- Attach a saline lock to the IO cannula, and then provide syringe boluses through the lock.

Step 9: Any drug or fluid that can be delivered to the patient by IV route can be equally given to the IO route which includes vasoactive drug infusions, such as epinephrine drip. Ensure that all medications should be accompanied with a saline flush.

- Use these guidelines to follow up the patient after establishing IO access. Note that Follow-ups are important.
- Monitor the site frequently for signs of swelling.
- Ensure to replace the IO access with vascular access within 24 hours. IO needles are designed for short term

use. Replacing IO needle with long-term vascular access is done in the intensive care unit.

- Administering fluids or drugs through displaces needle may lead to critical complications, such as tissue necrosis or compartment syndrome. So, ensure to supervise the needle to make sure it's not displaced.

ACUTE CORONARY

SYNDROMES

Right Ventricular Infarction

Patients suffering from inferior or right ventricular infarction often display excess parasympathetic tone. If parasympathetic is inappropriately discharge, it can cause symptomatic bradycardia and hypotension. If Hypotension is present, it's usually because of a combination of hypovolemia, which means decreased Left Ventricular filling pressure, and bradycardia.

- Deliver a normal solution of 250 to 500 mL to the patient and reassesses the patient.
- If the patient has improved a bit, and there's no sign of either volume overload or heart failure, repeat the saline administration up to 1 to 2L
- Volume administration may be key to saving patients with RV infarct and hypotension.

A slow heart is incorrect when hypotension is present. The heart rate should be faster when there's low blood pressure, this is because fluid bolus increases RV filling pressures which in turn causes increase in the strength of the RV contraction; this is called Starling Mechanism. The increased strength of the RV contraction would increase blood flow through to the lungs, and ultimately LV filling pressure and cardiac output.

Inferior MI with AV Block

A severe inferior wall myocardial infarction, which is commonly a right coronary artery problem, may lead to a symptomatic second-degree or third-degree AV block with a junctional and narrow-complex escape rhythm. There would be no need for transcutaneous pacing (TCP) and a transvenous pacemaker if the patient remains asymptomatic and hemodynamically stable. Nevertheless, the patient should be monitored and prepared for TCP if high-degree block occurs and the patient becomes suddenly becomes symptomatic or unstable before expert cardiology evaluation.

- AV block usually happen when there is excess vagal tone and atrioventricular nodal ischemia. The patient could remain stable if junctional pacemaker cells can function and maintain an adequate ventricular rate. This rhythm usually displays a narrow-complex QRS and a ventricular rate of about 40 to 50 beats per minute. The patient would remain stable, if a large amount of myocardium is nonfunctional or comorbid conditions exist.

- Use the Bradycardia algorithm, if the bradycardia is symptomatic
- Prepare the patient for TCP
- If the patient becomes symptomatic, use the atropine to increase both the blood pressure and the heartrate. The recommended initial atropine dose is 0.5 mg IV bolus. While making sure not to exceed 3 mg, repeat every 3 to 4 minutes. Don't go above the dose necessary to stabilize the patient because excess atropine may increase ischemia excessively increasing heart rate and contractility.
- If an unstable patient does not respond to atropine, then initiate TCP or infusion of chronotropic drug, such as epinephrine from 2 to 10 mcg per minute, or dopamine from 2 to 20 mcg/kg per minute. Deliver and titrate to patient response.
- If the patient is still unresponsive to drugs or TCP, start transvenous pacing.

Expert consultation is often needed for evaluation and recommendation of AV block with AMI as it can be pretty difficult to do. Recommendations include transvenous temporary pacemaker etc.

PRACTICAL QUESTIONS AND ANSWERS

1. The impact of Atropine on vagal reflexes is:

Answer: A lessening in Vegas reflexes as the ventricular crabbiness is expanded.

2. An impact of low portion of dopamine is:

Answer: Renal vasodilatation

3. Describe where the femoral reflex is found and its functions:

4. In ventricular fibrillation including a patient that didn't react to a few defibrillations or lidocaine, what is the necessary treatment?

5. Why are endotracheal tube stylets utilized?

Answer: Endotracheal tube stylets are utilized to make tubes structure fittings

6. Verapamil is what type of medication?

Answer: Verapamil is a calcium channel blocker

7. Propranolol is what kind of medication?

Answer: Propranolol is a beta-blocker

8. The mechanism of activity of adenosine on the heart is?

Answer: The component of activity of adenosine on the heart is the downturn of sinus node and AV node movement.

9. Are the statements below TRUE or FALSE?

While choosing a bag-valve mask device, a pop off valve is desirable.

While choosing a bag-valve mask device, the elements desirable consists of transparent mask, self-expanding bag and a non-breathing valve. In this manner,

Answer: The statements are FALSE.

10. Lidocaine might be deadly in what sort of rhythm?

Lidocaine might be deadly in idioventricular rhythm

11. Is the statement below TRUE or FALSE?

Utilization of systematic antibiotics ought to be utilized in preventing infectious complication of intravenous cannulas.

The utilization of systematic antibiotics ought not be utilized in the process to preventing infectious complications of intravenous cannulas. In this manner,

Answer: the statement is FALSE.

12. Is the statement below TRUE or FALSE?

Whenever the origin of a wide tachycardia is not known, verapamil ought to be utilized.

Verapamil should not be utilized when the beginning of a wide tachycardia is unknown, hence,

Answer: the statement is FALSE

13. Which medication depresses the siphoning capacity of the heart muscle in therapeutic doses?

Answer: Propranolol depresses the siphoning capacity of the hearth muscle in therapeutic doses.

14. An overdose of what should calcium chloride be thought of?

Answer: heart block.

15. During CPR, which if the following is the preferred vein for initial cannulation?

A.   external jugular vein

B.   femoral vein

C.   subclavian vein

D.   antecubital vein

Answer: Antecubital vein is the preferred vein during initial cannulation.

16. Which of the following is an exclusion of what traumatic injuries may include?

A.   cardiac tamponade

B.   hyperkalemia

C.   shock

D.   tension pneumothorax

Answer: Traumatic injuries may include all the listed options except hyperkalemia.

17. Which of the following treatments should be first used to treat ventricular fibrillation after initiating CPR?

A.   intubation

B.   defibrillation

C.   epinephrine IV

D.   lidocaine IV

Answer: Defibrillation

18. Is the statement below TRUE or FALSE?

Greater tidal volume is provided usually by mouth-to-mask compared to tidal volume provided by bag-valve mask devices.

Answer: TRUE

19. When performing endotracheal suction, should suction be applied?

Answer: Suction should be avoided while inserting the catheter.

20. Signs and symptoms of stroke include:

Answer: The signs and symptoms include confusion, photophobia, headache, nausea, vomiting, vertigo, hearing loss, change in vision and weakness.

21. What type of acidosis usually occur in an acute cardiac arrest?

Answer: Respiratory and metabolic acidosis are the types of acidosis that usually occur in acute cardiac arrest.

23. What is the primary function of a laryngoscope in intubation?

Answer: A laryngoscope's primary function is to visualize the vocal cords for proper endotracheal tube placement.

24. When is synchronized cardioversion indicated?

Answer: Synchronized cardioversion is indicated in hemodynamically unstable patients with supraventricular or ventricular tachycardias.

25. What is the first-line drug for acute symptomatic bradycardia?

Answer: Atropine is the first-line drug for acute symptomatic bradycardia.

26. What is the effect of epinephrine on peripheral vascular resistance?

Answer: Epinephrine increases peripheral vascular resistance by stimulating alpha-adrenergic receptors.

27. What does the mnemonic 'MONA' stand for in ACLS in myocardial infarction treatment?

Answer: 'MONA' stands for Morphine, Oxygen, Nitroglycerin, and Aspirin.

28. Which drug is contraindicated in cocaine-induced chest pain?

Answer: Beta-blockers are contraindicated in cocaine-induced chest pain due to the risk of unopposed alpha-adrenergic receptor activity.

29. What is the significance of capnography in ACLS?
Answer: Capnography is used to monitor CPR's effectiveness and detect spontaneous circulation (ROSC) return.

30. What is the preferred method for securing a definitive airway in cardiac arrest?
Answer: Endotracheal intubation is the preferred method for securing a definitive airway in cardiac arrest.

31. What is the initial dose of amiodarone for ventricular fibrillation or pulseless ventricular tachycardia?
Answer: The initial dose of amiodarone for VF or pulseless VT is 300 mg IV.

32. How does magnesium sulfate work in torsades de pointes?
Answer: Magnesium sulfate stabilizes cardiac membranes and can terminate torsades de pointes.

33. What are the indications for administering sodium bicarbonate in cardiac arrest?

148

Answer: Sodium bicarbonate is indicated in cardiac arrest with hyperkalemia, tricyclic antidepressant overdose, or pre-existing metabolic acidosis.

34. What is the role of targeted temperature management (TTM) in post-cardiac arrest care?

Answer: TTM is used to improve neurological outcomes by reducing brain injury in post-cardiac arrest patients.

35. What is the significance of a 'widened QRS complex' in ECG interpretation?

Answer: A widened QRS complex may indicate ventricular tachycardia or electrolyte imbalances.

36. What is the indication for using a non-rebreather mask in ACLS?

Answer: A non-rebreather mask is indicated for patients requiring high concentrations of oxygen.

37. What is the importance of the 'Chain of Survival' in ACLS?

Answer: The 'Chain of Survival' highlights key steps in cardiac arrest management to improve survival rates.

38. How does hyperventilation affect intrathoracic pressure during cardiac arrest?

Answer: Hyperventilation can increase intrathoracic pressure and decrease venous return, thus lowering cardiac output.

39. When is invasive hemodynamic monitoring considered in ACLS?

Answer: Invasive hemodynamic monitoring is considered in cases of refractory shock or when non-invasive methods are inadequate.

40. What is the most common side effect of nitroglycerin in the treatment of acute coronary syndrome?

Answer: The most common side effect of nitroglycerin is hypotension, often accompanied by a headache.

41. What is the role of a beta-blocker in acute myocardial infarction?

Answer: Beta-blockers decrease myocardial oxygen demand and can limit the infarct size in acute myocardial infarction.

42. What is the recommended compression-to-ventilation ratio in two-rescuer adult CPR?

Answer: The recommended compression-to-ventilation ratio in two-rescuer adult CPR is 30:2.

43. What is the primary action of a loop diuretic in heart failure management?

Answer: Loop diuretics reduce fluid overload by increasing urine output, thereby decreasing preload and improving symptoms of heart failure.

44. What is the significance of recognizing a 'STEMI' on an ECG in ACLS?

Answer: Recognizing an ST-Elevation Myocardial Infarction (STEMI) on an ECG indicates a need for urgent reperfusion therapy, typically through percutaneous coronary intervention (PCI).

45. What is the dose of magnesium sulfate for treating life-threatening ventricular arrhythmias?

Answer: For life-threatening ventricular arrhythmias, 1-2 grams of magnesium sulfate is administered IV over 5-20 minutes.

46. How does hypothermia affect the pharmacokinetics of medications used in cardiac arrest?

Answer: Hypothermia can slow the metabolism of drugs, leading to prolonged effects and increased risk of toxicity.

47. What is the significance of 'ROSC' in cardiac arrest management?

Answer: Return of Spontaneous Circulation (ROSC) signifies the restoration of a palpable pulse and is a critical goal in cardiac arrest resuscitation.

48. When is fibrinolytic therapy contraindicated in acute ischemic stroke?

Answer: Fibrinolytic therapy is contraindicated in acute ischemic stroke with a history of intracranial hemorrhage, recent major surgery, or uncontrolled hypertension.

49. What is the role of diltiazem in managing atrial fibrillation with rapid ventricular response?

Answer: Diltiazem, a calcium channel blocker, is needed to slow the ventricular rate in atrial fibrillation with rapid ventricular response.

50. How is hypovolemia addressed in the ACLS algorithm?

Answer: The ACLS algorithm addresses hypovolemia by administering IV fluids to improve circulation and cardiac output.

51. What is the significance of the AVPU scale in assessing a patient's level of consciousness?

Answer: The AVPU scale (Alert, Verbal response, Painful response, Unresponsive) is used to assess a patient's level of consciousness quickly.

52. What are the criteria for advanced airway placement during CPR in ACLS?

Answer: Advanced airway placement during CPR is considered for prolonged resuscitation efforts when bag-mask ventilation is ineffective or if there is a risk of aspiration.

53. What is the role of norepinephrine in treating septic shock?

Answer: Norepinephrine is a first-line vasopressor to increase pressure and perfusion in septic shock.

54. How does synchronized cardioversion differ from defibrillation?

Answer: Synchronized cardioversion delivers a shock timed with the R-wave of the ECG, while defibrillation delivers an unsynchronized shock.

55. What is the primary goal of using vasopressors in cardiac arrest?

Answer: The primary goal of vasopressors in cardiac arrest is to increase coronary and cerebral perfusion pressure during CPR.

56. When is a Valsalva maneuver indicated in ACLS?
Answer: The Valsalva maneuver is indicated to terminate supraventricular tachycardia (SVT) by increasing intrathoracic pressure and stimulating the vagus nerve.

57. What are the key signs of tension pneumothorax in a cardiac arrest patient?
Answer: Key signs of tension pneumothorax include unilateral absence of breath sounds, distended neck veins, and tracheal deviation.

58. What is the preferred route of drug administration during cardiac arrest?
Answer: During cardiac arrest, the preferred route of drug administration is intravenous (IV) or intraosseous (IO) if IV access is not available.

59. How does pulse oximetry assist in managing a critically ill patient?

Answer: Pulse oximetry provides continuous monitoring of oxygen saturation, which is essential for assessing respiratory function and guiding oxygen therapy.

60. What is the primary indication for the use of glucagon in ACLS?

Answer: Glucagon is used in ACLS for beta-blocker or calcium channel blocker overdose when conventional treatments are ineffective.

61. What is the role of therapeutic hypothermia in post-cardiac arrest care?

Answer: Therapeutic hypothermia is used to lower body temperature to protect the brain and improve neurological outcomes in post-cardiac arrest patients.

62. In ACLS, what is the significance of a 'peaked T-wave' on an ECG?

Answer: A peaked T-wave on an ECG may indicate hyperkalemia, a critical electrolyte disturbance that requires prompt treatment.

63. What is the preferred treatment for stable ventricular tachycardia?

Answer: Amiodarone is the preferred treatment for stable ventricular tachycardia, especially if the patient has underlying heart disease.

64. How does aspirin function in managing acute coronary syndrome (ACS)?

Answer: Aspirin acts as an antiplatelet agent, reducing blood clot formation and decreasing the risk of heart attack or stroke in ACS.

65. What is the significance of measuring end-tidal CO_2 in cardiac arrest?

Answer: End-tidal CO_2 measurement helps assess CPR's effectiveness and can provide an early indication of ROSC.

66. In what situation is the use of a cricothyroidotomy indicated in ACLS?

Answer: Cricothyroidotomy is indicated when other forms of airway management, like intubation, are impossible or have failed in a cannot-intubate-cannot-oxygenate scenario.

67. What is the initial management strategy for symptomatic bradycardia?

Answer: The initial management strategy for symptomatic bradycardia includes the administration of atropine, and if ineffective, pacing or epinephrine may be considered.

68. When are inotropic agents used in the ACLS setting?

Answer: Inotropic agents are used in the ACLS setting for managing patients with cardiogenic shock or severe heart failure where there is diminished cardiac output.

69. What is the role of a precordial thump in cardiac arrest?

Answer: A precordial thump can be attempted as an immediate response in witnessed, monitored, unstable ventricular tachycardia or ventricular fibrillation without defibrillation equipment.

70. In ACLS, how is a suspected opioid overdose managed?

Answer: Suspected opioid overdose is managed with supportive care and the administration of naloxone, an opioid antagonist.

71. What is the primary indication for administering sodium bicarbonate during CPR?

Answer: Sodium bicarbonate is primarily administered during CPR for known pre-existing hyperkalemia or in cases of tricyclic antidepressant overdose.

72. How is a tension pneumothorax treated in the emergency setting?

Answer: Treatment of tension pneumothorax involves the immediate decompression of the chest cavity, typically by needle thoracotomy followed by chest tube placement.

73. What is the importance of obtaining a 12-lead ECG in acute coronary syndrome?

Answer: A 12-lead ECG is important in acute coronary syndrome for diagnosing the type and extent of myocardial infarction and guiding treatment decisions.

74. What is the role of vasodilators in acute heart failure management?

Answer: Vasodilators, like nitroglycerin, reduce cardiac preload and afterload, easing the work of the heart in acute heart failure.

75. When is mechanical ventilation indicated in ACLS?

Answer: Mechanical ventilation is indicated in cases of respiratory failure, severe hypoxemia, or protective airway strategies are needed in comatose patients.

76. How is a flail chest managed in the prehospital or emergency setting?

Answer: Flail chest is managed with pain control, ensuring adequate ventilation, and in severe cases, may require mechanical ventilation.

77. What are the indications for using a pacemaker in bradycardia management?

Answer: Indications for a pacemaker in bradycardia include symptomatic bradycardia unresponsive to medical therapy, certain types of heart block, and bradycardia-induced syncope.

78. What is the significance of 'bag-valve mask' ventilation in emergency care?

Answer: Bag-valve mask ventilation is critical for providing effective ventilation to apneic patients with inadequate respiratory effort.

79. In ACLS, what is the purpose of sequential bilateral arm compressions in pulmonary embolism?

Answer: Sequential bilateral arm compressions in pulmonary embolism aim to increase venous return and cardiac output in a massive PE where CPR is ineffective.

80. What is the first step in managing a patient with a suspected stroke in the emergency department?

Answer: The first step in managing a suspected stroke is a rapid assessment to determine the onset of symptoms and perform a focused neurological exam.

81. How does lidocaine function as an antiarrhythmic in cardiac emergencies?

Answer: Lidocaine functions as a sodium channel blocker, stabilizing myocardial cell membranes and treating ventricular arrhythmias.

82. What is the importance of early recognition and treatment of sepsis in ACLS?

Answer: Early recognition and treatment of sepsis are vital to prevent the progression of septic shock and organ dysfunction and improve survival outcomes.

83. What role does epinephrine play in anaphylactic shock management?

Answer: Epinephrine is the first-line treatment in anaphylactic shock, reversing airway constriction and improving circulation.

84. How is hyperkalemia managed in the setting of cardiac arrest?

Answer: Management of cardiac arrest with hyperkalemia includes administering calcium, insulin with glucose, and sodium bicarbonate to stabilize cardiac membranes and shift potassium intracellularly.

85. When is a chest X-ray essential in assessing a cardiac arrest patient?

Answer: A chest X-ray is essential post-resuscitation to assess for possible causes of cardiac arrest, such as pneumothorax or pulmonary edema.

86. What is the significance of a 'shockable rhythm' in ACLS?

Answer: A 'shockable rhythm' in ACLS refers to ventricular fibrillation or pulseless ventricular tachycardia, treated with immediate defibrillation.

87. How does a beta-blocker reduce mortality in post-myocardial infarction patients?

Answer: Beta-blockers reduce mortality post-MI by decreasing myocardial oxygen demand, reducing arrhythmias, and preventing adverse cardiac remodeling.

88. What is the purpose of using a bougie in endotracheal intubation?

Answer: A bougie is used as a guide during difficult endotracheal intubation to facilitate the placement of the endotracheal tube.

89. In ACLS, how are electrolyte imbalances, like hypomagnesemia, managed in cardiac arrest?

Answer: Hypomagnesemia in cardiac arrest is managed by administering magnesium sulfate, which can help stabilize cardiac rhythms.

90. What is the role of bedside ultrasound in ACLS?

Answer: Bedside ultrasound can be used in ACLS to quickly identify reversible causes of cardiac arrest, such as pericardial effusion or ventricular dysfunction.

91. What considerations are important when selecting an IV fluid type for resuscitation?

Answer: When selecting an IV fluid for resuscitation, considerations include the patient's electrolyte balance, acid-base status, and presence of heart failure or renal impairment.

92. How does proper head positioning aid in effective bag-valve-mask ventilation?

Answer: Proper head positioning, such as the sniffing position, opens the airway and improves the effectiveness of bag-valve-mask ventilation.

93. What is the significance of a 'non-shockable rhythm' in cardiac arrest?

Answer: A 'non-shockable rhythm' in cardiac arrest, such as asystole or pulseless electrical activity, requires CPR and pharmacological interventions instead of defibrillation.

94. When is intraosseous (IO) access preferred over intravenous (IV) access in emergency care?

Answer: IO access is preferred when IV access is difficult or time-consuming to establish, especially in cardiac arrest or critically ill patients.

95. How do glucocorticoids assist in managing acute exacerbations of COPD or asthma?

Answer: Glucocorticoids reduce inflammation and airway edema in acute exacerbations of COPD or asthma, improving breathing.

96. What is the rationale behind the use of therapeutic hypothermia in cardiac arrest?

Answer: Therapeutic hypothermia is used post-cardiac arrest to reduce neurological damage by slowing metabolic rates and protecting against ischemic injury.

97. How is acute right ventricular failure managed in the situation of a massive pulmonary embolism?

Answer: Acute right ventricular failure in massive pulmonary embolism is managed with hemodynamic support, anticoagulation, and, in some cases, thrombolytic therapy.

98. What are the indications for performing a pericardiocentesis in cardiac emergencies?

Answer: Pericardiocentesis is indicated in cases of cardiac tamponade, where fluid accumulation in the pericardium impairs heart function.

99. When is dopamine used as a first-line vasopressor in shock management?

Answer: Dopamine is used as a first-line vasopressor in shock, particularly in patients with signs of low cardiac output and poor perfusion.

100. How is cardiac asthma differentiated from pulmonary asthma in an emergency setting?

Answer: Cardiac asthma, caused by heart failure, is differentiated from pulmonary asthma by assessing for associated symptoms like orthopnea, paroxysmal nocturnal dyspnea, and fluid overload signs.

AFTERWORDS

As you approach the Advanced Cardiac Life Support (ACLS) certification, you prepare not just for an exam but also to become a lifeguard in the most crucial situations. The path you are about to embark on is one of great responsibility and enormous reward.

Remember that obtaining ACLS certification entails more than technical abilities and medical understanding. It's a path to becoming more capable, confident, and compassionate healthcare professionals. Each chapter you read, scenario you practice, and talent you learn puts you closer to being someone's hero in their hour of need.

You are about to learn how to navigate the turbulent waters of cardiac emergencies, restore peace and order amid mayhem, and, most significantly, give someone the gift of a second shot at life. This information is potent and comes with the responsibility of using it wisely and skillfully.

Do not be intimidated by the trials that lie ahead. Accept them. Perseverance and dedication are required on the path to mastery. Remember why you started whenever you feel overwhelmed. You've come to make a difference, to save lives, and to be the oasis of calm amid a storm.

The ACLS certification is more than just a badge of honor; it demonstrates your dedication to providing excellent patient care. It acknowledges your capacity to execute under pressure, quickly make key decisions, and confidently lead.

Take pride in your study as you prepare for this test. Be happy for your victories, learn from your mistakes, and always keep sight of your ultimate aim. Your path to ACLS certification is as much about personal development as professional development.

And when that day arrives, know that you have earned more than just a degree but also the respect and trust of those you will serve. You are not merely passing a test but becoming a light in the darkest times.

So, study hard, train hard, and have faith in yourself. The journey may be difficult, but the prize is precious. Your greatest accomplishments will be the lives you rescue and the difference you create.

Finally, I wish you the best of luck on your ACLS certification path. May it be a rewarding, illuminating, and inspirational experience. More heroes like you are needed in the world.

Thank you for reading this far. And if you have the moment, kindly leave your honest review if you find the book useful. This will help us know what to improve on and other readers will know what to expect.

Thank you again dear reader, and we hope you find other titles from us useful as you progress.